DIAGNOSTIC PI(

CW00961715

Ortho~~peedics~~

Lipmann Kessel MBE (MLTY), MC, FRCS
Previously, Emeritus Professor of Orthopaedics,
University of London, England

Uta F Boundy
Chief Medical Photographer
Institute of Orthopaedics,
Royal National Orthopaedic Hospital,
London and Stanmore, Middlesex

M Wolfe

Titles published in the Diagnostic Picture Tests series include:
DPT in Cardiology
DPT in Clinical Medicine, Vol 1–4
DPT in Clinical Neurology
DPT in Dermatology
DPT in Endocrinology
DPT in Gastroenterology
DPT in General Medicine
DPT in General Surgery
DPT in Infectious Diseases
DPT in Injury in Sport
DPT in Ophthalmology
DPT in Paediatrics, 2nd edn
DPT in Rheumatology
DPT in Urology

Copyright © L. Kessel & U.F. Boundy, 1988
Published in 1988 by Wolfe Medical Publications Ltd,
Printed by Hazell Books Ltd, Aylesbury, England
ISBN 0 7234 0900 5
Reprinted 1990 and in 1993 by Wolfe Publishing, an imprint of
Mosby–Year Book Europe Limited

For full details of all Mosby–Year Book Europe Limited titles
please write to Mosby–Year Book Europe Limited, Lynton
House, 7–12 Tavistock Square, London WC1H 9LB, England.

A CIP catalogue record for this book is available from the British
Library.

Preface

By taking up this book you have shown an interest in Orthopaedics. Our aim is to stimulate that interest. Whether you are students—undergraduates or postgraduates—or general practitioners, we have tried to illustrate for you as many orthopaedic conditions as possible in this compact format. Keep it with you, use it as a handy reference when faced with some of the not-so-often-encountered disorders and, most important, do not stop the 'Question Game' when you reach the last page.

A word of explanation is necessary. In using the plural I am attempting to speak for the late Professor Lipmann Kessel who, of course, is the main author of this book. Many readers will be familiar with the work of this most excellent of orthopaedic surgeons and I am not the only person who sadly misses his inspiring presence since his untimely death in June 1986.

I should like to thank my colleague, Mr. Dirk DeCamp, for often holding the fort while L.K. and I were busy in the preparation of this, his last publication. To his memory goes my dedication.

Uta F. Boundy

Acknowledgements

We would like to thank members of the consultant staff, Royal National Orthopaedic Hospital, London and the Institute of Orthopaedics, London, jointly and severally for their permission to use illustrations of patients under their care.

Dedication

It is my wish to dedicate this book to the late Peter Wolfe, Publisher, who died on 22nd December 1986: in memory of the Author, the late Lipmann Kessel, Emeritus Professor of Orthopaedics who died on 5th June the same year.

Beryl Kessel

1 A two-year-old child with 'bandy legs' who was otherwise normal.
(a) What is the diagnosis?
(b) What is the differential diagnosis?

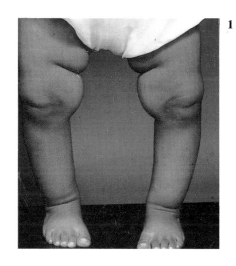

2 The left hand of an elderly lady.
(a) What is the diagnosis?
(b) What is the 'tumour' on the radial aspect of her index finger?

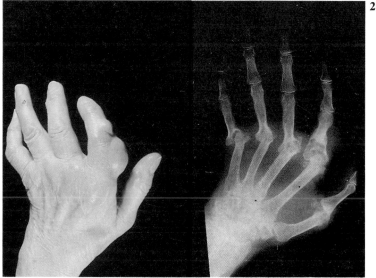

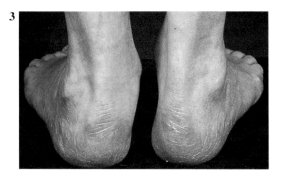

3 A young man suffered multiple injuries in a road traffic accident. Several months later he had a painful heel which was broadened and valgus. What is the diagnosis?

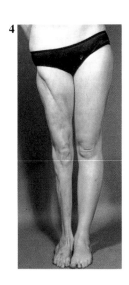

4 A young woman showed extensive soft-tissue deformation in her right thigh and generalised muscle-wasting in her right leg, which is shorter than the left. The radiographs were normal and there were no associated lesions elsewhere.
(a) What was the diagnosis?
(b) How would you establish it?

5 The hand of a patient suffering from rheumatoid polyarthritis; gradual deformation of the fingers has developed.
(a) What is this deformation called?
(b) How is it brought about?

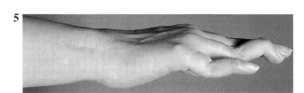

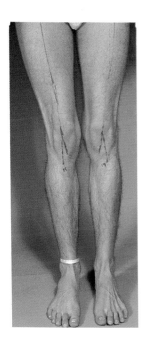

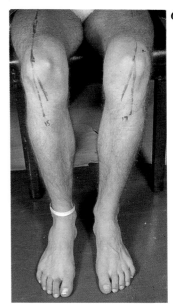

6 A young man presents with troublesome knees; his patellae keep 'slipping out of place'.
(a) What is this condition?
(b) What is its aetiology?
(c) How do you measure the 'q-angle' and why is it so called?

7 A child born with a deformity below the left knee; the leg is bowed backwards and the foot held in a marked dorsiflexion.
(a) What is the diagnosis?
(b) What is the differential diagnosis?

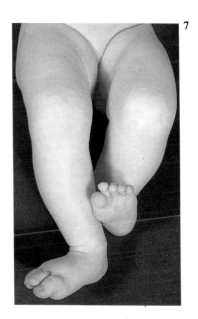

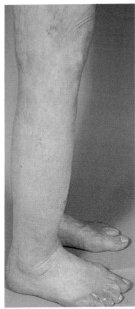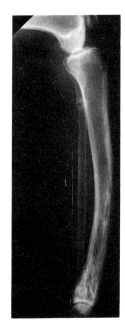

8 The leg of a 60-year-old man.
(a) What is the diagnosis?
(b) To what do you attribute the anterior bowing of the tibia?

9 The feet of mother and daughter.
(a) Name the abnormality.
(b) What is its official designation?

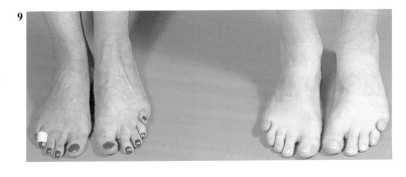

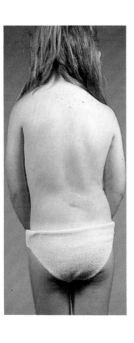

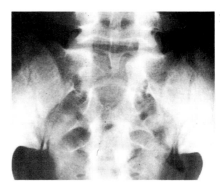

10 A six-year-old child's lumbar spine shows slight deformation with a notable dimple and hyperaemic patch. The shoulders are at different levels, the left scapula being higher than the right. What is the diagnosis?

11 This child has suffered from partial paralysis of her right arm since birth.
(a) What is this condition?
(b) To what is it due?

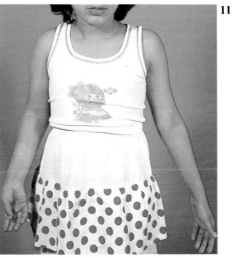

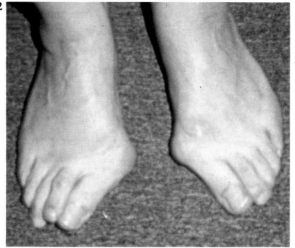

12 An old lady shows very broad forefeet with marked 'bunions'. No other joints are involved.
(a) What is the basic deformity?
(b) How is it classified?
(c) What is a bunion?

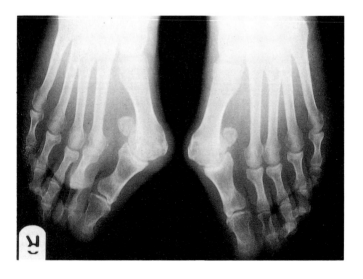

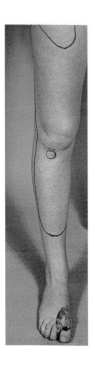

13 The right leg of a young woman complaining of numbness in the marked areas above and below the knee. A small patch is visible in the prepatellar region and another at the base of her 1st and 2nd toes. A tumour was removed from her pelvis before she developed the anaesthesia. Which nerve has been affected?

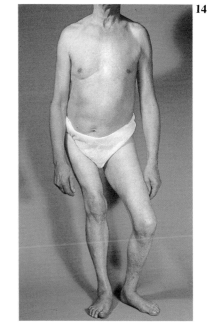

14 When standing this young man cannot straighten his left leg—the knee stays in flexion; the radiograph shows a marked increase of the lumbar lordosis.
(a) What is the condition?
(b) What is the primarily affected joint?

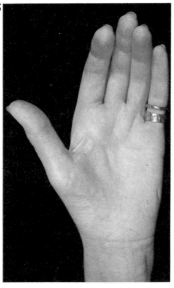
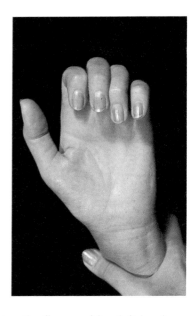

15 This patient cannot fully straighten the fingers of her left hand; on wrist extension her fingers become strongly flexed into the hand.
(a) What is this sign called?
(b) To what is it attributed?

16 A young man showing absence of the normal lumbar lordosis and marked transverse creases in the skin and fat across both loins; this appearance is typical.
(a) What is the diagnosis?
(b) What would you expect to see on the radiographs?

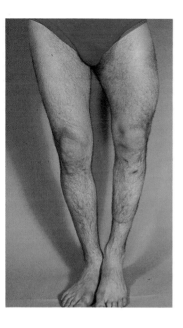 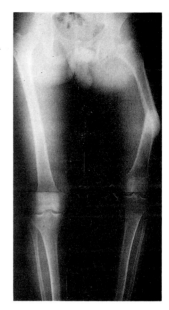

17 The legs of a young man who was involved in a motorcycle accident five years previously. There were no clinical abnormalities other than shortening and bowing of the left femur. What is the diagnosis?

18 A woman suffering from rheumatoid arthritis was treated with Benoxaprofen. Her thumbnails show signs of disease.
(a) Name the condition.
(b) Is it attributable to the disease or to the treatment?

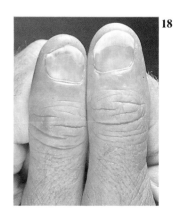

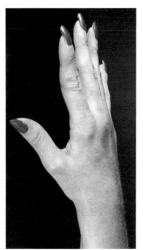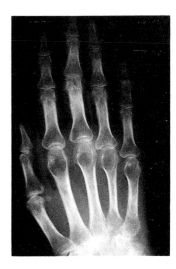

19 The right hand and wrist of a middle-aged woman.
(a) What is the diagnosis?
(b) What is the deformity of the index finger?
(c) To what is the deformity due?

20 This man has pain in his left shoulder. *All* modalities of movement are grossly limited and he has to assist his left arm into internal rotation with his right. The radiograph shows multiple 'classical' loose bodies. What is the diagnosis?

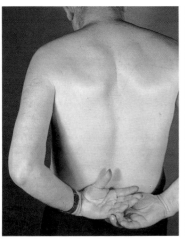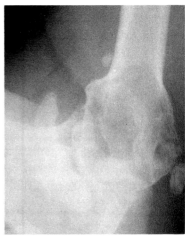

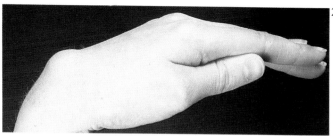

21 What is the slightly painful swelling on the dorsum of the wrist of a young woman? It is firm but not bone-hard and is not tender. It is best seen with the wrist fully flexed.

22 A young man was brought in by his mother because his chest 'looks funny'. Plain radiographs reveal no abnormalities.
(a) What is the nature of this condition and what is its importance?
(b) How should it be treated?

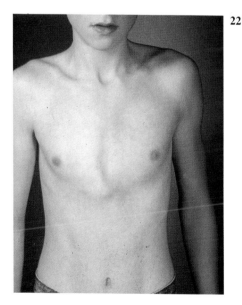

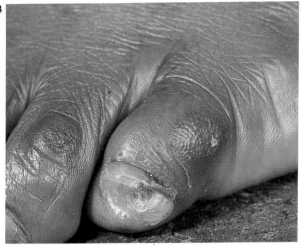

23 The foot of a West African patient showing a small lump on the little toe with a circular constriction at its base and deformation of the nail. What is the diagnosis?

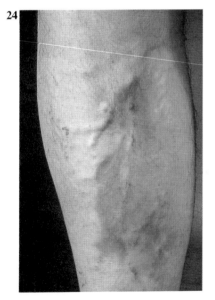

24 The leg of a lady suffering from diabetes. The skin over her shin is markedly hyperaemic, tender and swollen. What is the condition?

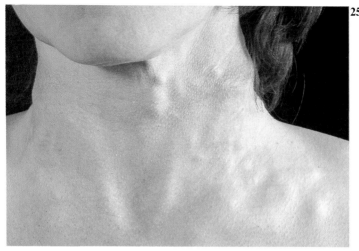

25 Photograph and chest radiograph of a middle-aged woman showing multiple masses, some of which can be felt; some are pigmented, others not. Note particularly the soft tissue mass at the apex of the right lung, just below the first rib. Give a possible diagnosis.

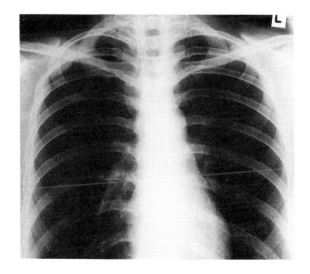

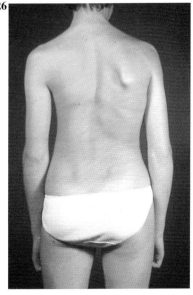

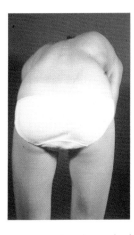

26 A young man showing spinal curvature.
(a) What is the diagnosis?
(b) What simple clinical test is required to determine further management and treatment?

27 Examination of the hips of an elderly man. A radiograph shows loss of joint space on the right, and minor alteration of trabeculation of the neck of femur, so-called 'primary osteo-arthritis'.
(a) What is this clinical test?
(b) What is its purpose?

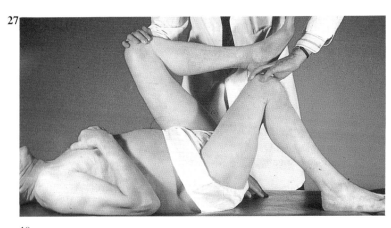

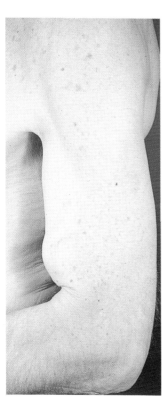

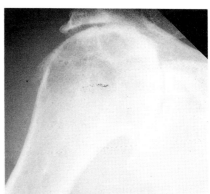

28 The lump on the front of the arm is painless.
(a) What does the radiograph show?
(b) What is the diagnosis?

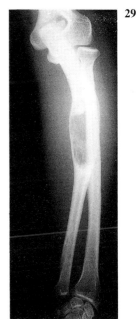

29 Radiograph of the forearm of a 40-year-old woman with a painless swelling on the ulnar aspect: full investigations showed no abnormality.
(a) What is the diagnosis?
(b) What treatment can be proposed?

30

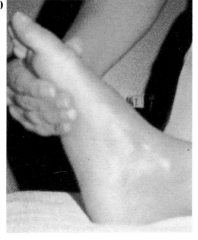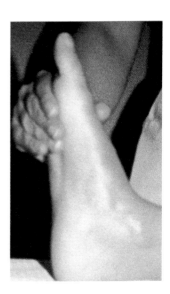

30 The feet of a young woman who has had an operation, as shown in the radiograph. She suffered from anterior poliomyelitis as a child.
(a) What operation has been performed and by what eponym is it known?
(b) What is its principal indication?

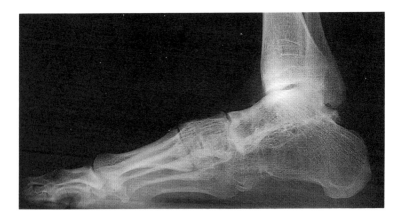

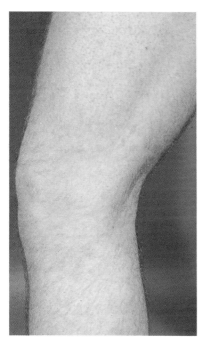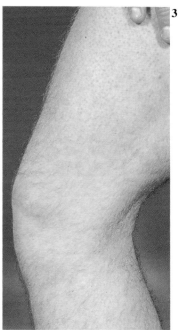

31 A young man suffered severe injury to his right knee some years ago; he now complains of an unstable knee that gives way without warning.
(a) What sign can be observed?
(b) To what may it be ascribed?

32 The hand of a 55-year-old mechanic.
(a) What is the diagnosis?
(b) What particular questions should be asked?

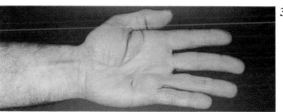

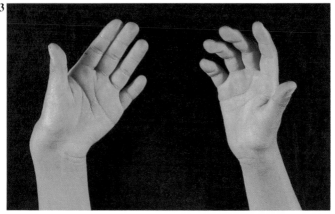

33 The wrists of a young boy showing marked deformity on the left. There are no other clinical signs. The radiograph shows that the carpal bones—only on the radial side—are disorganised. What is the diagnosis?

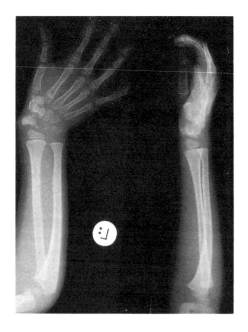

34 A man suffered a fractured leg and was treated in his village by bandaging and splinting. What effects on the leg can be seen?

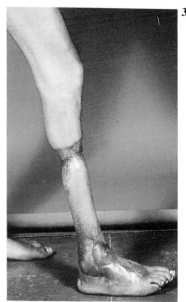
34

35 This teenage girl is dwarfed and has deformed legs; her intelligence is above average.
(a) Give a possible diagnosis.
(b) What is the differential diagnosis?
(c) What other investigations should be made?

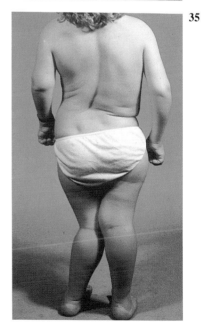
35

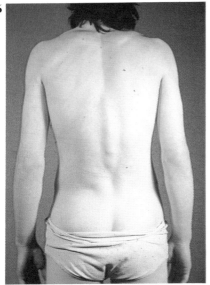 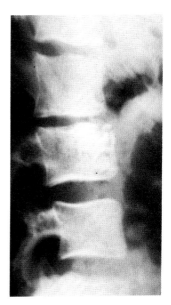

36 An otherwise normal and healthy young man shows slight prominence of the dorsolumbar region of the spine; he has absolutely full and painless movement.
(a) What is the diagnosis?
(b) What is the differential diagnosis?
(c) What further investigation may be required?

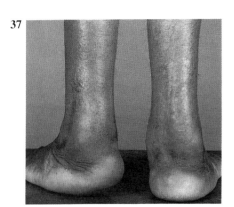

37 A teenager born with deformed feet; he has had several operations.
(a) What is the nature of the deformity of the left foot?
(b) What operation has been performed on the right foot?

38 This one-year-old has had a weak and deformed arm since birth.
(a) What is the diagnosis?
(b) To what is the deformity attributed?

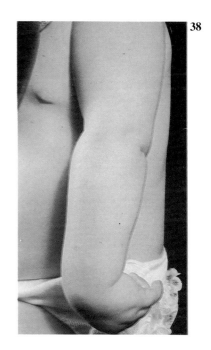

39 A teenager has scoliosis which is not obliterated on forward flexion. How is this condition classified?

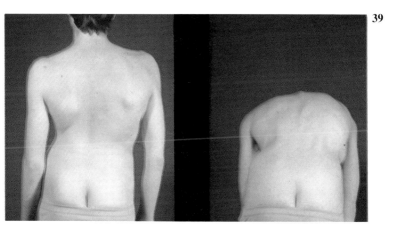

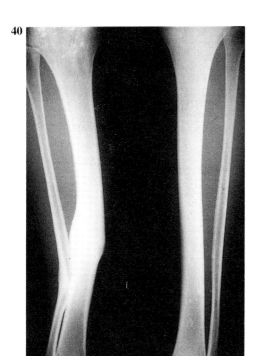

40 Anteroposterior and lateral radiographs showing malunion of the fractured tibia and fibula of a man who was involved in an accident two years earlier.

(a) What is the deformity?

(b) Is further investigation required?

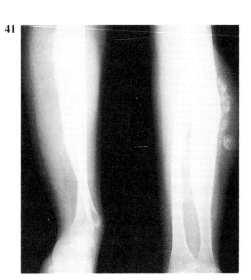

41 Plain radiographs of the right forearm of a young woman who presented with a recurring swelling; a tumour had been excised previously.

(a) What is the diagnosis?

(b) What is the differential diagnosis?

(c) Are further investigations required?

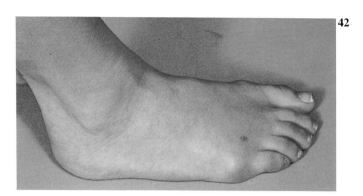

42 The foot of a young woman showing a swelling on the outer aspect.
(a) What is the diagnosis?
(b) What is the cause of the swelling?

43 This teenager's back is collapsed sideways and forwards, as can be seen by the deep crease in her loin; she is unable to sit up straight. The appearance is characteristic. What is the diagnosis?

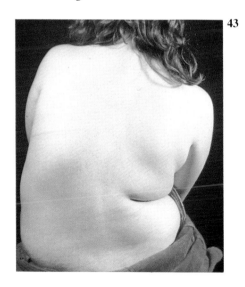

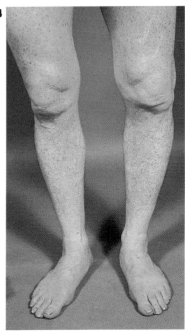

44 The knees of a 60-year-old man taken while weight-bearing, five years after an accident; the deformity can be passively corrected.
(a) What is the diagnosis?
(b) What is the cause of the condition?

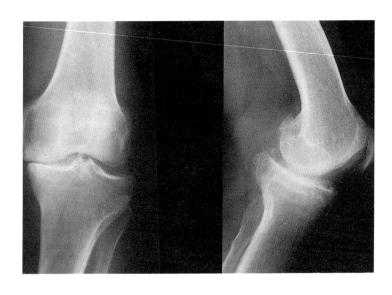

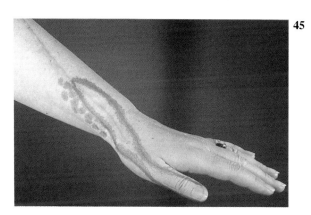

45 The outlined area shows loss of skin-sensibility following an operation for de Quervain's disease. What has happened?

46 The right knee of a middle-aged woman who has had an operation in childhood.
(a) What is this condition?
(b) How did it develop?

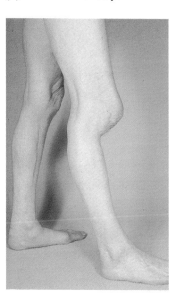

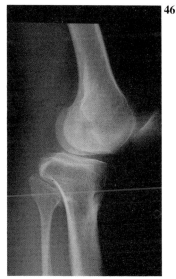

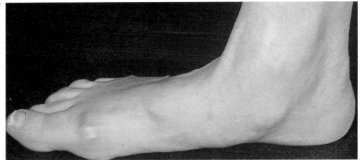

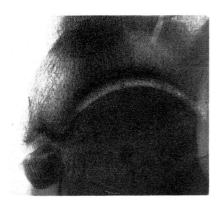

47 The foot of a 35-year-old man who complains that his shoe is rubbing on the prominent lump shown.
(a) What is the condition?
(b) What is the cause?

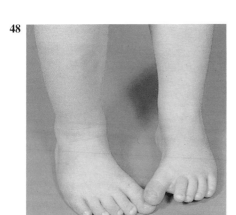

48 An 18-month-old child walks with his feet turned inwards. There is full passive movement of all joints and no paralysis.
(a) How would you classify this condition?
(b) What is the treatment?

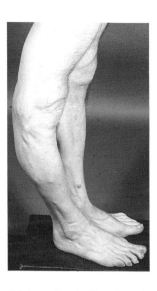 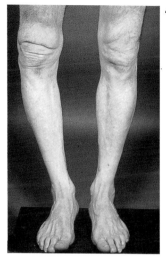

49 A patient suffered major injury to his right knee several years previously.
(a) How should the deformity be classified?
(b) What is the cause?

50 The feet of a young woman who has already had a simple 'bunionectomy' on her right foot.
(a) What is the deformity affecting her lesser toes.
(b) What investigations should be performed?

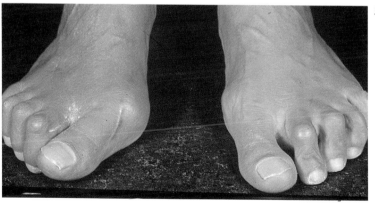

51

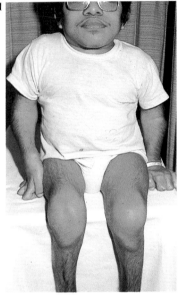 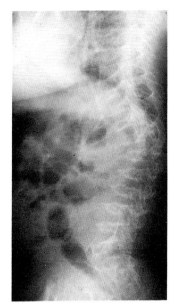

51 A 14-year-old boy could only stand with difficulty; a lateral radiograph of his spine is shown; skeletal survey showed widespread dysostosis. He was of normal intelligence but suffered from corneal opacities and deafness.
(a) What is this condition?
(b) To which metabolic abnormality may it be ascribed?

52 The feet of a 65-year-old man, weight-bearing; there is no muscle paralysis.
(a) What is the deformity?
(b) What additional information is required?

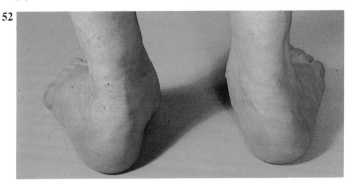

53 A young woman with severe knock-knees. Radiographs of her hands and wrists are shown.
(a) What is the diagnosis?
(b) Are further investigations required?

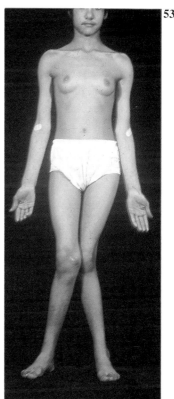

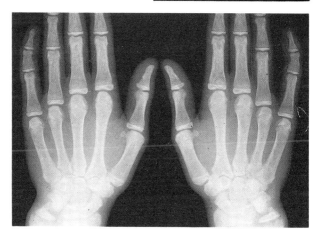

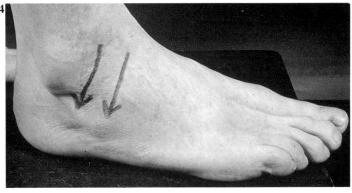

54 A 'dumb-bell' soft tissue tumour on the outer aspect of the ankle. It is hard but semi-fluctuant.
(a) What is the diagnosis?
(b) Why is the tumour thus shaped?

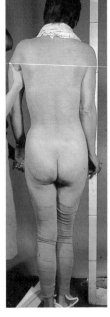

55 This woman suffers from severe 'lumbago-sciatica'.
(a) What clinical sign can be observed in her back?
(b) What would you expect to find on straight-leg-raise testing?
(c) What do these signs and symptoms indicate?
(d) What procedure is required to establish the diagnosis?

56 This patient was involved in a severe motor accident some years earlier. The marked skin area shows alteration of sensibility. Red cross-hatching—total loss of sensation; Black cross-hatching—partial loss of sensation. Muscle weakness was evident below the knee. A radiograph of her pelvis is shown.
(a) What is the diagnosis?
(b) Comment on the manifestations of the injury.

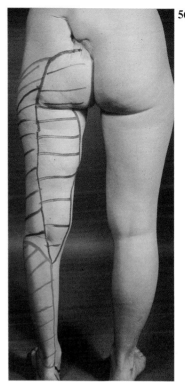

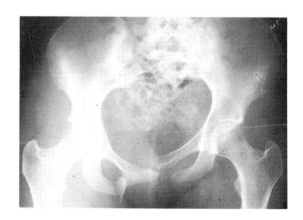

57

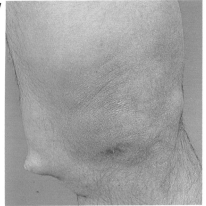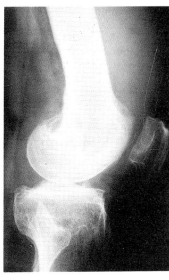

57 The knee of a 35-year-old man showing complex soft tissue swelling. He is generally healthy, no other joints are involved and all serological investigations were normal.
(a) What is the diagnosis?
(b) How can it be established?

58 The nails of a man who suffers from polyarthritis. What is the diagnosis?

58

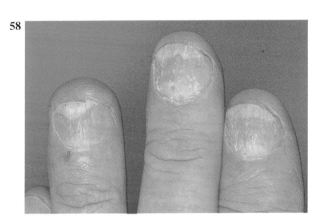

59 The face and skull radiograph of a 65-year-old man; the appearance of both is characteristic.
(a) What is the diagnosis?
(b) What are the other common orthopaedic manifestations of this condition?

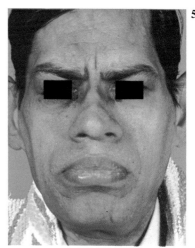

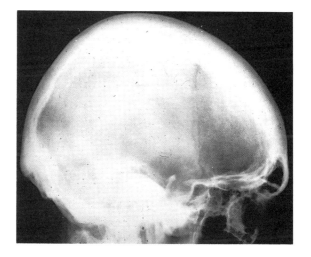

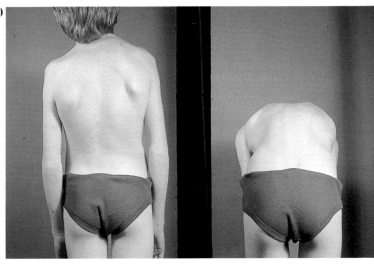

60 The spine of a 15-year-old boy.
(a) What is the diagnosis?
(b) Which features enable you to name and classify this condition?

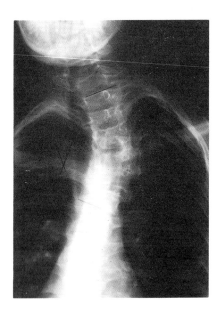

61 A 22-year-old patient had sudden onset of severe pain in the right knee. The swelling was partly due to synovial thickening and partly to increased joint fluid. There had been no injury. General examination showed only inflammation of one eye. The radiographs were non-contributory.
(a) What is the diagnosis?
(b) How can it be established?

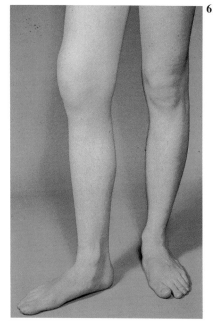

62 Multilocular soft tissue swellings on the dorsum of several fingers. With what condition may these swellings be associated?

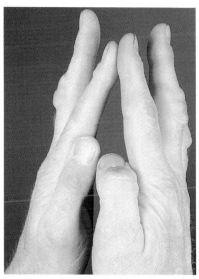

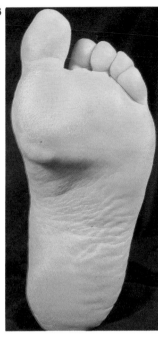

63 (a) What is the deformity seen on the foot of a 20-year-old woman?
(b) What may be the cause?
(c) What other investigations are required for diagnosis?

64 A knock-knee deformity in a generally healthy 3-year-old boy; radiographs were non-contributory. The same boy is shown at 9 years old.
(a) What is the most probable diagnosis?
(b) What is the prognosis?

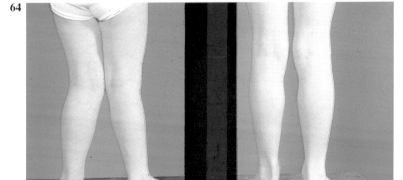

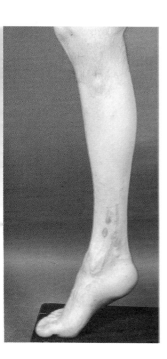 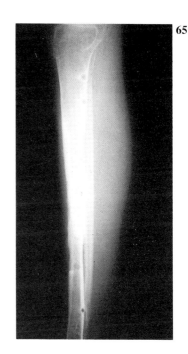

65 The leg of a young man who suffered a severe football injury two years previously. The ankle deformity cannot be passively corrected.
(a) What is the diagnosis?
(b) What are the diagnostic features?

66 Name the condition seen in the right foot of a ten-year-old boy.

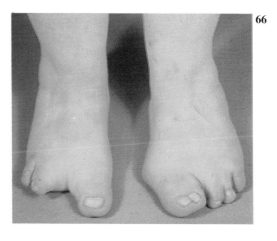

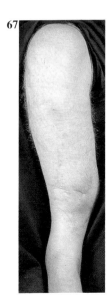 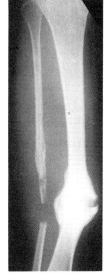

67 The leg of a man who suffered severe fractures of his right tibia and fibula 4 years earlier.
(a) What is the diagnosis now?
(b) Can you reconstruct the history since injury?

68 A middle-aged woman had poliomyelitis in infancy. She had several operations on her hindfoot; her forefoot shows an obvious residual deformity, which is mobile.
(a) What is the deformity?
(b) What is its cause?

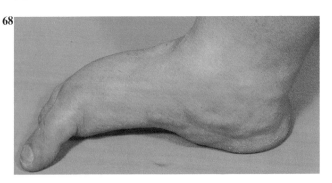

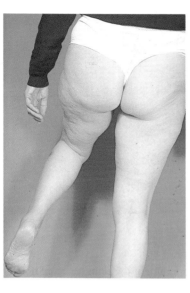 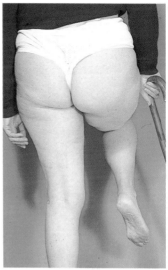

69 A patient standing first on one leg, then on the other. Her right leg bears weight easily, and the left hip is seen to rise—note the level of the buttock creases. She cannot stand on her left leg without the aid of a stick—the right buttock is seen to droop.
(a) What is this clinical test?
(b) What does it reveal?

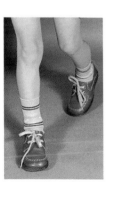 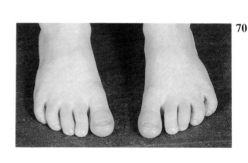

70 A child walks 'pigeon-toed'.
(a) To what may this condition be ascribed?
(b) What advice or treatment could be offered?

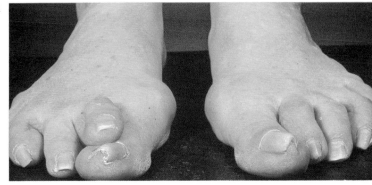

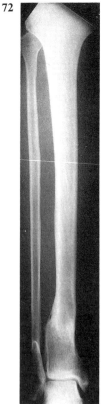

71 (a) What deformities are apparent in the feet of this middle aged woman.
(b) How do they occur?

72 Lateral radiograph of the right tibia and fibula of a young man who suffered a fracture just above the ankle.
(a) Has he any residual deformity?
(b) If so, what is its nature?

73 A young woman complains of pain and instability of her left knee. The mass on its antero-lateral aspect is mobile. What is the diagnosis?

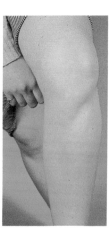

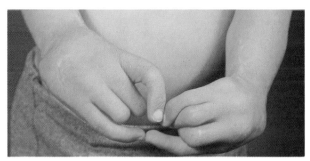

74 The forearms and hands of this young man have been deformed since birth.
(a) What is the condition?
(b) What are its principal features?

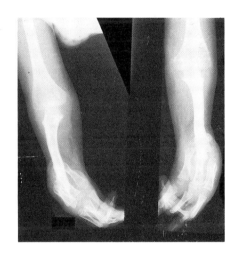

75 (a) What striking clinical sign is shown?
(b) What are the possible causes?

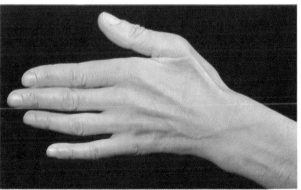

76

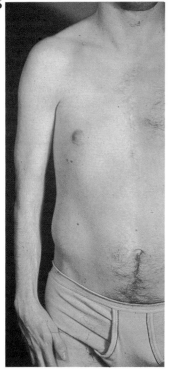
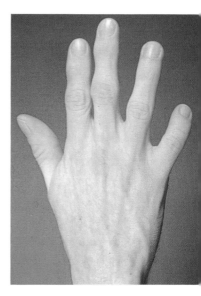

76 What is the rare syndrome shown in this young man's chest and right hand?

77 Both feet of this young teenager show a very similar deformity. Note particularly the bilateral high arches and the extended big toes which indicate spasticity. He suffered from petit mal following measles in infancy.
(a) What is the differential diagnosis?
(b) Where is the neurological lesion likely to be?

77

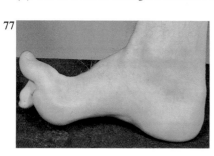

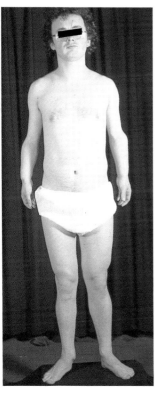
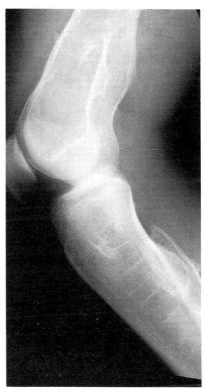

78 A young man of below normal stature but above average intelligence; a typical radiograph from his skeletal survey is shown.
(a) What is the condition?
(b) What is the typical clinical—as distinct from radiological—feature?

79 This man is trying to hunch his shoulders; there is an operation scar in the right anterior triangle of the neck.
(a) What is the diagnosis?
(b) How has the condition arisen?

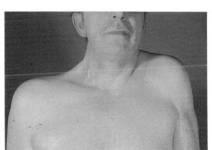

80

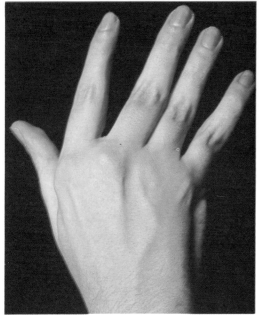

80 A patient is being treated for rheumatoid arthritis of the hands. What is the cause of the rash?

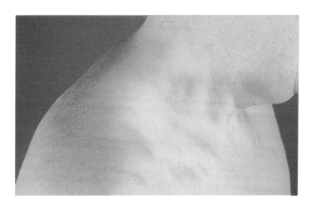

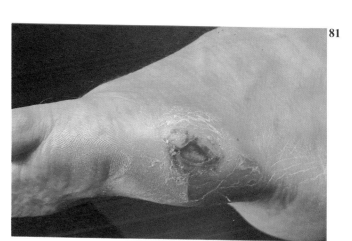

81 An indolent sore on the outer side of a patient's left foot.
(a) What are the possible underlying causes?
(b) What action must be taken?

82 The right hand of a man who had a crush injury without skin loss three months previously.
(a) What is the diagnosis?
(b) On which features is it based?

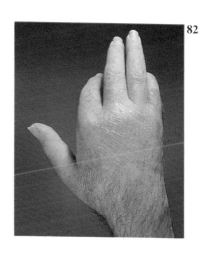

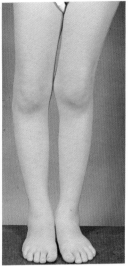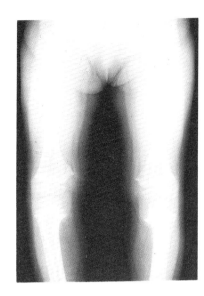

83 (a) What is the deformity of the knees seen in this girl?
(b) What are the principal features of the radiograph?
(c) Suggest how this condition should be classified.

84 This patient was asked to turn both arms outwards. From his expression, he is making a strong effort to do so. No abnormal neurological signs or symptoms are present. What is a likely diagnosis?

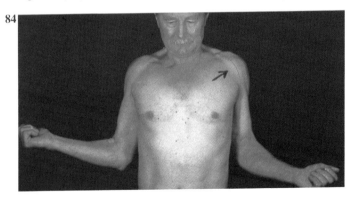

85 At least two of this patient's interphalangeal joints are severely afflicted. The diagnosis was in doubt until a lesion appeared in the skin overlying the distal interphalangeal joint of the index finger.
(a) What is the diagnosis?
(b) What investigations are required to confirm it?

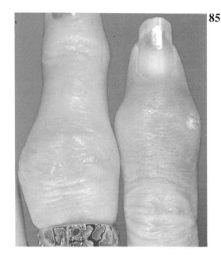

86 Following a motorcycle accident this young man had loss of sensibility in his right hand—as shown by marking. One eyelid is drooping and the pupil is small.
(a) What is the pathology?
(b) What is the syndrome?

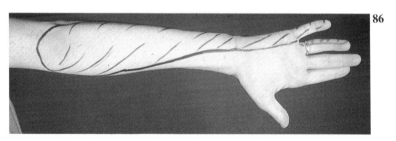

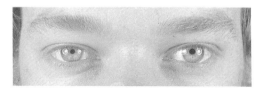

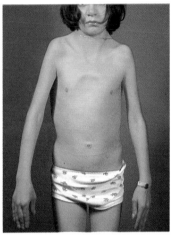

87 This girl has a deformed chest and a slightly elevated shoulder, but no pain.
(a) How would you classify her condition?
(b) What treatment is recommended?

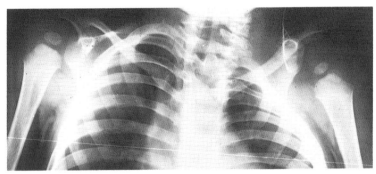

88 This young woman cannot fully turn her head. What features suggest an exact diagnosis?

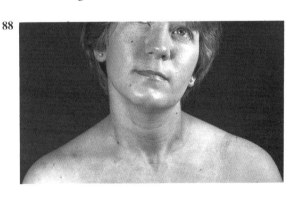

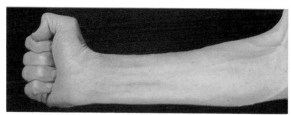

89 On contracting his elbow this man exhibits a powerful band that can be seen and felt underneath the skin on the antero-medial aspect of the joint.
(a) Name and describe the condition.
(b) What symptoms arise and what treatment is required?

90 An elderly man shows marked deformity of the feet.
(a) What is the likely diagnosis?
(b) Which features form the basis for the diagnosis?
(c) What serious associated disorders may be present in this condition?

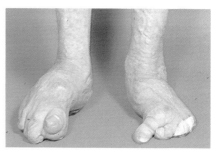

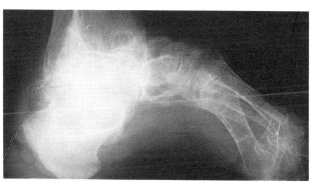

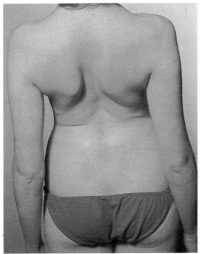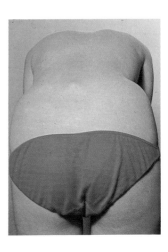

91 This young woman complains of backache. Forward flexion is full and free, but extension is severely limited. Note the marked creasing on either side of the lumbar spine, and an obvious prominence at the lumbosacral level.
(a) Can a diagnosis be made from this clinical evidence?
(b) What would you expect to find on a radiograph?

92 The several obvious masses on this sole are soft and fluctuant and give the impression of communicating with each other.
(a) What is the probable diagnosis?
(b) What tests or investigations will be required to confirm it?

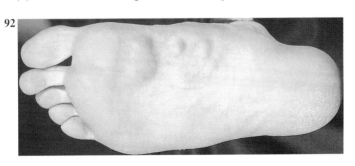

93 A middle-aged woman has a huge swelling of the calf which exhibits fluctuation. Radiographs of her wrists are also shown.

(a) What is the swelling and what is its nature?

(b) With what systemic condition is it associated?

(c) What is a radiograph of her knee likely to show?

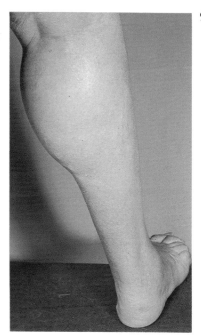

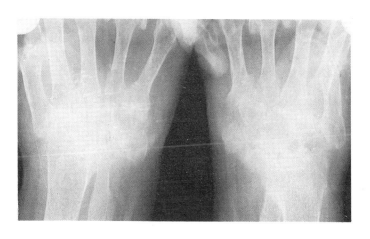

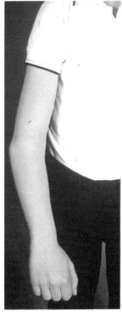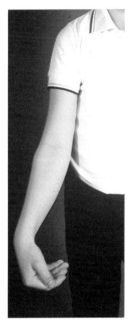

94 A young boy is shown trying to pronate and supinate his right forearm. Although pronation seems to be full, he is rotating his shoulder to achieve it. There is no history of injury. What is the diagnosis?

95 This child was born with deformed feet.
(a) What is the residual deformity of the left foot?
(b) What is it commonly called?
(c) What is the derivation of the *precise* clinical description?

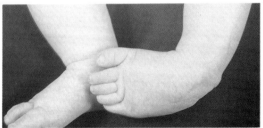

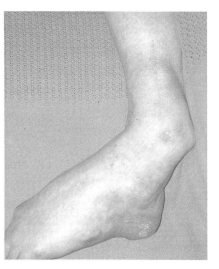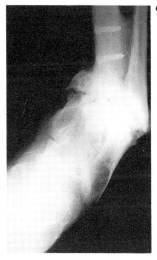

96 Five years after a serious motorcycle injury this patient's leg is passively mobile at the level of maximal deformity.
(a) What is the precise diagnosis?
(b) What is the likely history?

97 The hands of a patient suffering from rheumatoid polyarthritis show several typical abnormal features.
(a) What is the principal deformity?
(b) What is the cause?

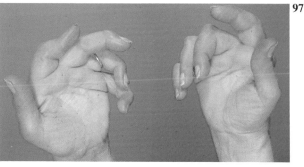

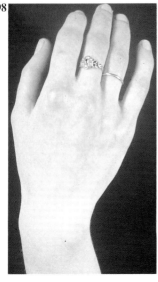

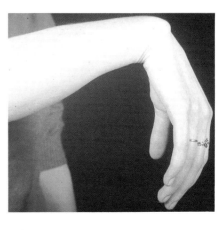

98 There is no history of injury to this patient's wrist.
(a) What is the deformity?
(b) How does it develop?

99 The legs of this girl were deformed at birth.
(a) Describe the clinical abnormalities.
(b) What is the diagnosis?
(c) What investigations would assist in establishing the diagnosis?

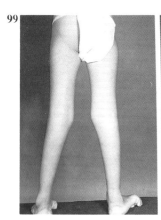

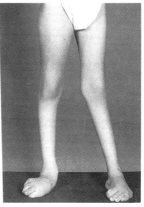

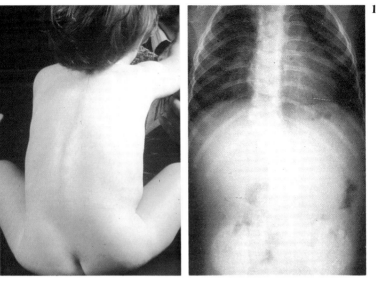

100 This child has a deformity of the lumbar spinal region; the normal lumbar lordosis is obliterated and lateral curvature is present. How would you classify this condition?

101 A patient has pain in his shoulder in the range of movement shown. What is the probable cause?

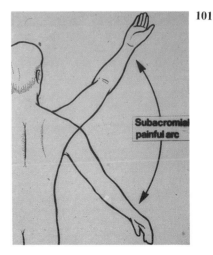

Subacromial painful arc

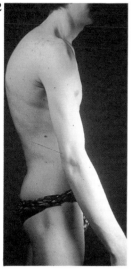 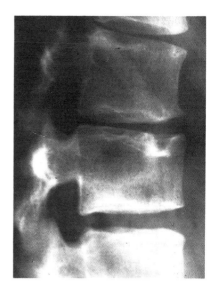

102 A 17-year-old boy with apparently powerful chest development complained of backache.
(a) What is the diagnosis?
(b) From what has it to be distinguished?
(c) What investigations are required?

103 The left hand of a middle-aged man. Note the deformity of the skin in the palm in the line of the ring finger.
(a) What is this lesion?
(b) What other clinical features assist diagnosis?

104 A baby undergoing treatment for congenital dislocation of the hip; the radiograph was taken when she attended for review.

(a) What is the abnormality, as seen on the radiograph?

(b) What observations would you make to the mother?

(c) What is the future management?

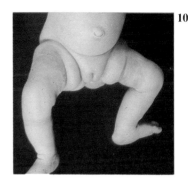

104

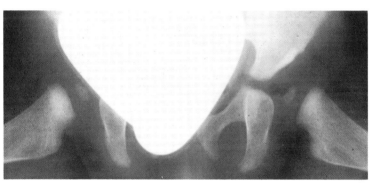

105 This 18-year-old girl complained that she 'has always been a bit lop-sided'. Examination showed a difference between the two sides of her upper chest and a higher right than left shoulder level. There were no other abnormal physical signs; radiographs were normal.

(a) What is the diagnosis?

(b) How can it be demonstrated?

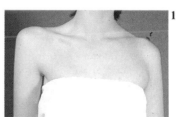

105

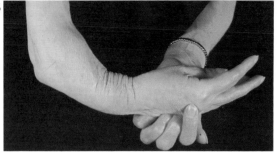

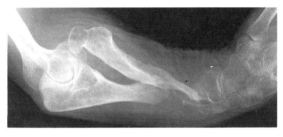

106 This old lady's forearm simply flops about unless it is held in the other hand; the condition has persisted since childhood despite many surgical interventions. What is the diagnosis?

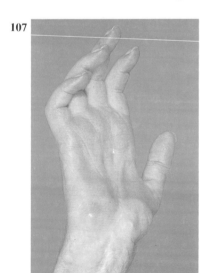

107 This man sustained an open injury to his right forearm several months earlier; there was widespread loss of sensibility in virtually all the front of his hand and fingers.
(a) What abnormal features are shown?
(b) What is the diagnosis and what may be deduced about the nature of the injury?

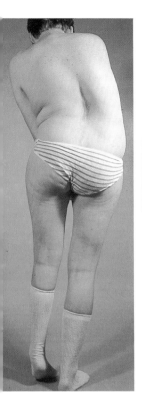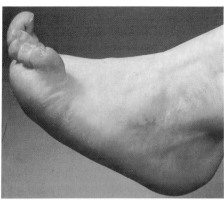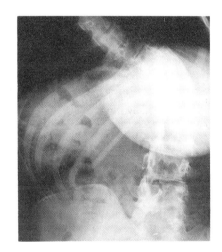

108 (a) What abnormal signs are seen in the lumbar spine and foot?
(b) What abnormality is shown on the radiograph?
(c) What is the diagnosis?

63

109

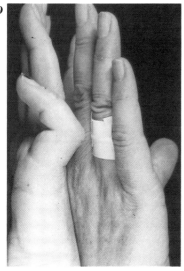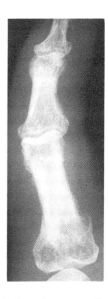

109 A patient damaged her right hand several weeks before these records were made. An apparently trivial fracture through the base of the proximal phalanx is seen on the radiograph. To what may the considerable deformity of her little finger be ascribed?

110

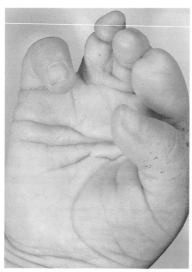

110 The hand of a child born with gross finger deformities; the ring finger looks as though it had been constricted by an intra-uterine band while the index finger seems to be amputated near its tip.
(a) What is the likely cause of these abnormalities?
(b) How should the diagnosis be confirmed?

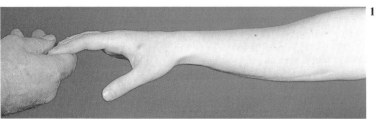

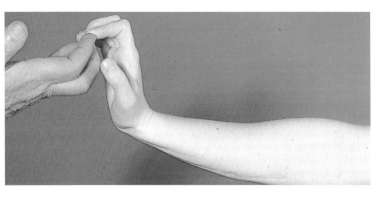

111 The right forearm and hand of a patient who suffered severe injury, including fractures, some years earlier. When the wrist is held straight or slightly flexed, the fingers are virtually straight; when the wrist is dorsiflexed, the fingers are pulled into powerful flexion.
(a) What is this sign and how is it produced?
(b) What is the basic traumatic anatomy?

112 A 16-year-old with a drooping right shoulder whose right scapula was correspondingly lower than the left. The radiographs showed a minimal cervicodorsal scoliosis.
(a) What clinical tests should be made?
(b) What is the probable diagnosis?

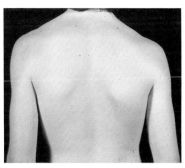

113

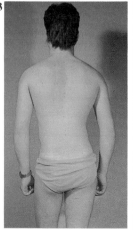 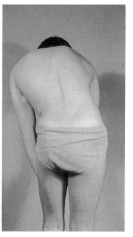

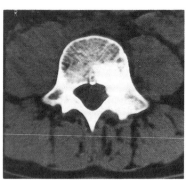

113 A young man complained of intense 'lumbago' on forward flexion; there was marked scoliosis of the pattern usually seen in 'sciatic scoliosis'. He had no severe leg pain and no abnormal neurological signs. The plain radiographs revealed no abnormality except for a slight increase in density on one side of the pedicle of L4, seen on the CAT scan. What is the diagnosis and differential diagnosis?

114

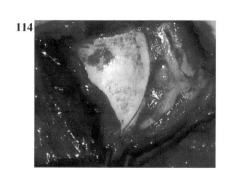

114 What is the lesion shown at operation on a patient diagnosed as having chronic rupture of the rotator cuff?

115 This 11-year-old girl of normal intelligence developed gradual bowing of her legs. Her physical development was rather below normal; radiographs were required as part of a skeletal survey.
(a) What is the diagnosis?
(b) What further investigations are needed to confirm the diagnosis?

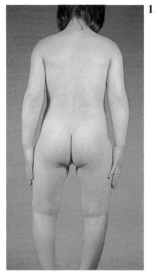

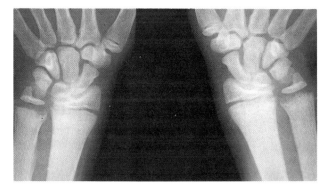

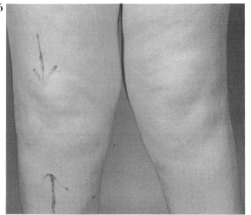

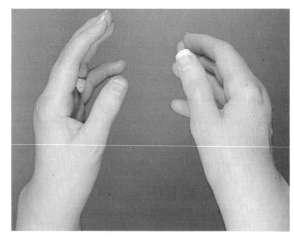

116 A 42-year-old woman complained of widespread aches and pains, swollen joints and malaise.
(a) What is the probable diagnosis?
(b) What investigations are required?

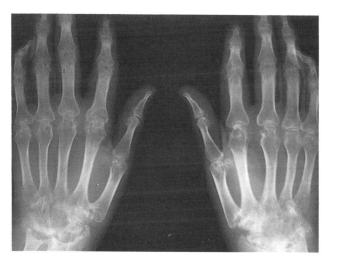

117 This 9-year-old girl presented with spinal deformity; she was born prematurely, and her educational progress was very slow. She had an abnormally small head-circumference and tended to hold her mouth open. Her family history suggested a degree of consanguinity of her parents.

(a) What is a possible diagnosis?
(b) What investigations are required?

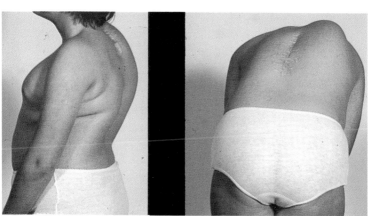

118

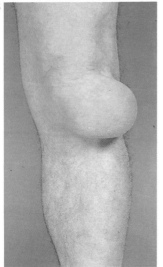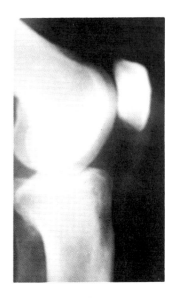

118 (a) What is the large mass in the patellar region of this left knee?
(b) In what way does the radiograph assist diagnosis?
(c) What are the differential diagnoses?

119 A patient involved in a road traffic accident was struck heavily on the right shoulder by a car; there is a painful hard swelling in the front of his chest. What is the diagnosis?

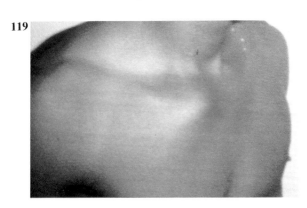

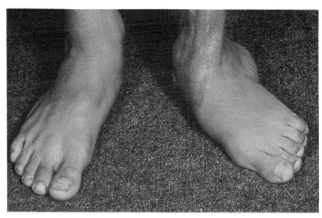

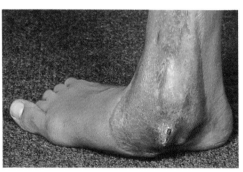

120 The left foot of a young man who had been run over by a motorcar. All soft tissues in the medial aspect of the lower leg and ankle were completely erased and subsequently have been covered by skingraft. The foot has become very deformed but the radiographs are, surprisingly, normal in all respects.
(a) What is the deformity?
(b) How has it developed?

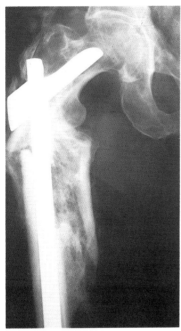

121 Radiograph of a severely comminuted fracture of the upper third of the right femur treated by internal fixation.
(a) What is this device called?
(b) What is the principal use?

122 The right hand of a man who suffered a crushing injury and cannot now straighten his fingers, particularly the middle one. Why?

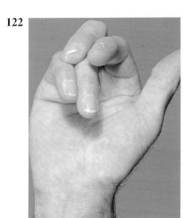
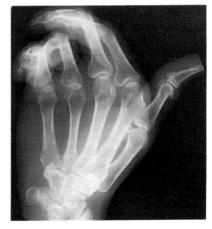

123 A 30-year-old man injured his knee ten years previously. There is a tense firm swelling on the outer aspect just below the level of the joint, most prominent in the position shown — flexed to 30°.
(a) What is the diagnosis?
(b) What are the differential diagnoses?

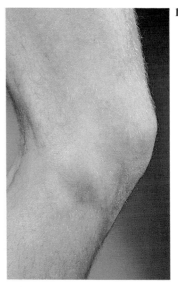

124 This boy complained of aching in his feet. Describe the abnormalities shown.

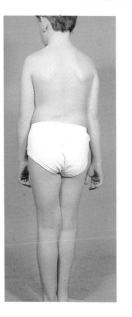

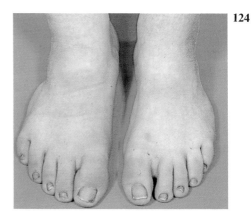

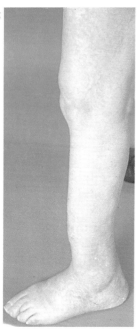

125 The left leg of an elderly lady who had an accident one year earlier. What is the diagnosis?

126 (a) What is the deformity of the foot in this 19-year-old girl?
(b) What investigations are required to make a full diagnosis?

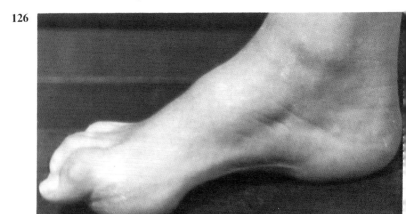

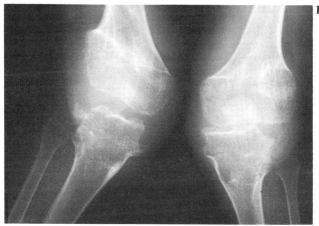

127 Radiograph of the knees of a 14-year-old boy who is of short stature and has a scoliosis. What investigations are required to differentiate between: rickets, old Still's disease, metaphyseal dysostosis or any other condition?

128 This man had chronic backache and marked limitation of movement; the full extent of his lateral and forward spinal flexion is shown.
(a) What is the probable diagnosis?
(b) What investigations should be performed?

128

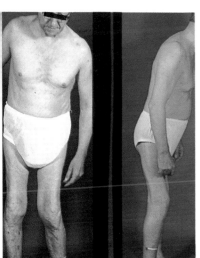
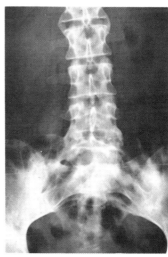

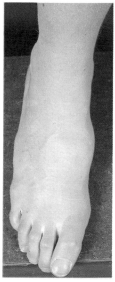 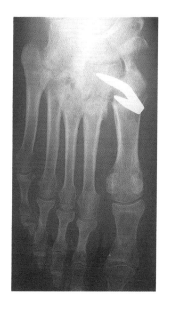

129 The right foot of a woman who suffered a severe injury which required manipulation. She later presented with pain and swelling, and required a further operation—subsequent radiograph is shown. What is the probable nature of the original injury?

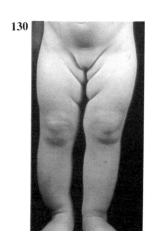

130 An 18-month-old girl presents with a bowed right leg. Note any other lesion which could assist in diagnosis.
(a) Describe the deformity precisely and any other visible abnormality.
(b) What is the diagnosis?
(c) What is the prognosis?

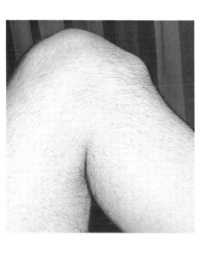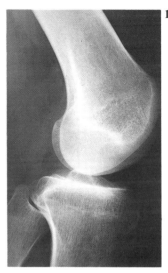

131 A 25-year-old man complained of a bony lump in the front of his knee; it is seen best in the flexed position. What is the diagnosis?

132 A middle-aged woman complained of weakness in her left hand.
(a) What clinical sign is evident?
(b) What is the likely cause?

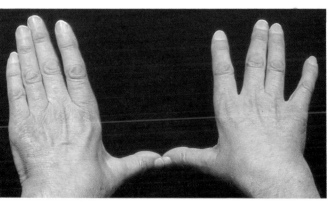

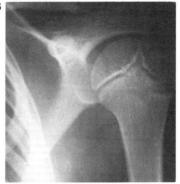

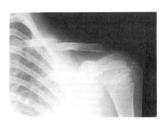

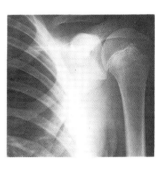

133 Serial radiographs of the left shoulder of a young man who first injured his clavicle at 9 years of age; he had a second injury at 13 years. What is the probable diagnosis?

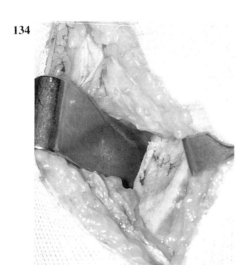

134 At operation, this lesion was disclosed on the lateral condyle of the femur of a young man who suffered from instability of his knee coupled with effusion. What is the diagnosis?

135 Lateral meniscus, removed from the right knee of a footballer after injury. Name the lesion.

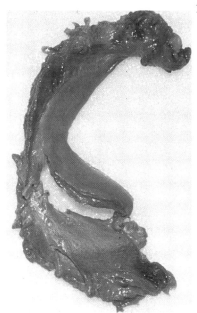

136 This 3-year-old's sister required an operation for severe knock-knees. The radiographs are normal.
(a) What is the diagnosis?
(b) Are follow-up examinations needed?
(c) What precise measurements should be made to determine progress?

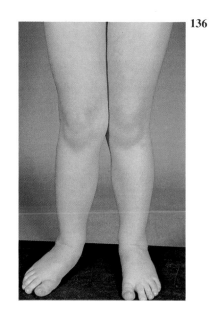

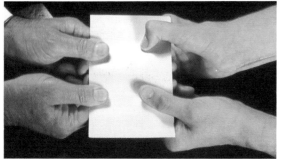

137 A patient complaining of weakness of his right hand is asked to grasp a card held by the examiner; note that the interphalangeal joint of his right thumb collapses into flexion.
(a) What is this test called?
(b) What is it intended to reveal?
(c) Why does the thumb collapse?

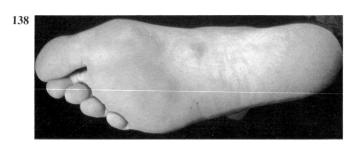

138 A tender nodule on the sole of a patient's right foot; it was firm and solid. What is the diagnosis?

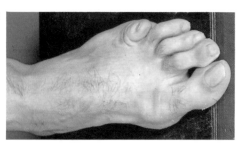

139 What deformities of the toes are seen?

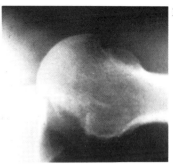

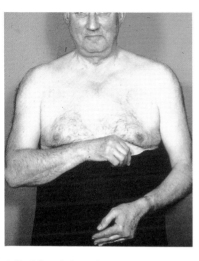

140 After injury in a motor accident the right shoulder is held in full internal rotation.
(a) What is the diagnosis?
(b) How does the X-ray assist diagnosis?

141 A young man constantly wore a ring on his left little finger; it became so tight it had to be removed under anaesthesia. He is shown trying to fully extend and fully flex the finger.
(a) What clinical abnormalities can be seen?
(b) What is the underlying pathology?

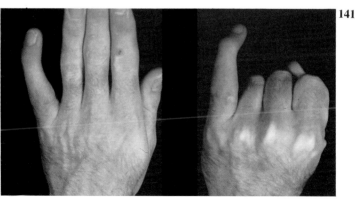
141

142

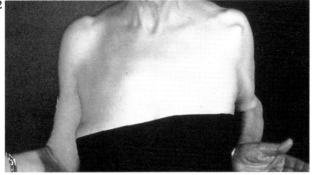

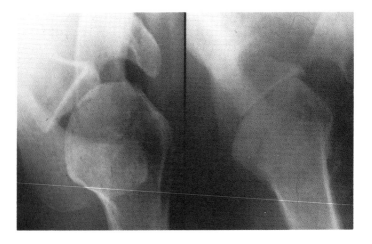

142 This patient has a flail left shoulder. Note the discoloration of her left hand, which was burned when accidentally immersed in hot water. Radiographs were taken at a six-month interval.
(a) What is the diagnosis?
(b) How would it be confirmed?

143 A 16-year-old girl whose patellae have been outlined. She had pain and was suspected of suffering from chondromalacia. Arthrography revealed no abnormality.
(a) What is the condition?
(b) To what may it be attributed?

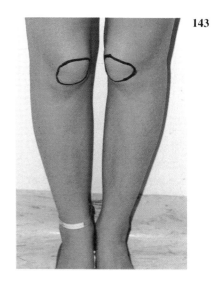

143

144 A 20-year-old patient complained of pain in both feet.
(a) What principal clinical sign may be anticipated on examination?
(b) What is the diagnosis?

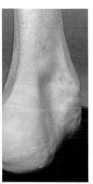
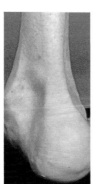
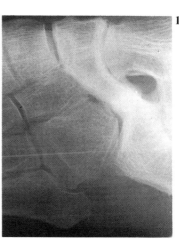

144

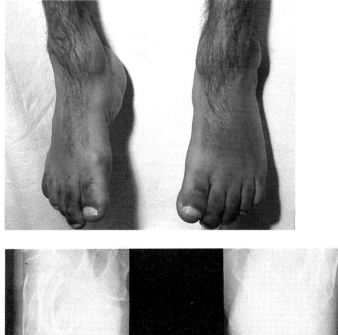

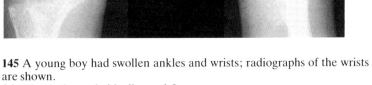

145 A young boy had swollen ankles and wrists; radiographs of the wrists are shown.
(a) What is the probable diagnosis?
(b) What investigations should be performed to establish the diagnosis?

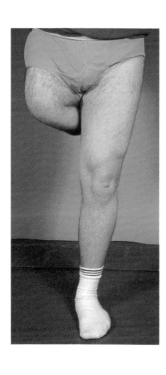

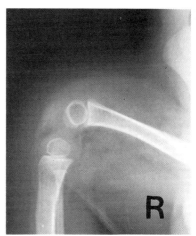

146 A young man was born with a very short right lower limb.
(a) What is the diagnosis?
(b) What are the features of this condition?

147 A 3-year-old has unequal leg-lengths. Are there any other signs which suggest a diagnosis?

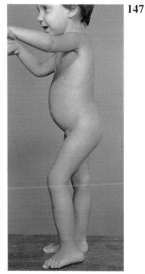

148

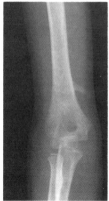

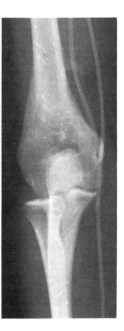

148 A girl complained of pain in her forearm when typing; the plain film shows an exostosis pointing forwards.
(a) What does the exostosis represent and what is the diagnosis?
(b) What does the brachial arteriograph show and what would you expect to find at operation?

149 A painful swelling of this patient's thumb gradually developed over the year after she had pricked herself while sewing. The radiograph was non-contributory. What is the probable diagnosis?

149

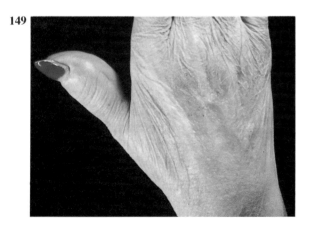

150 A small tumour was removed from within the median nerve of a patient who had a painful swelling in the forearm. Pressure caused tingling in her thumb and index finger.
(a) What is the diagnosis?
(b) What are the principal features of this tumour?

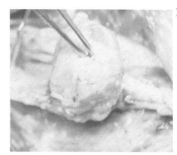

151 Radiographs of the hips of a young man who originally presented at 14 years of age.
(a) What is the diagnosis?
(b) What clinical signs would you have expected at 14 years of age?
(c) What changes are apparent after an interval of 7 years?

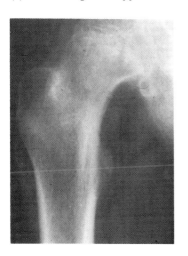
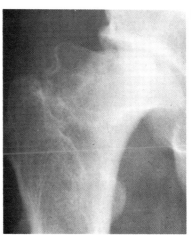

152

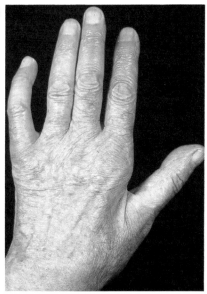

152 The left hand of a middle-aged woman complaining of weakness of grip; she also admitted to some numbness of the skin of the little finger. There is no history of injury.
(a) What abnormal signs are present?
(b) What is the probable diagnosis?
(c) Why is it so called?

153

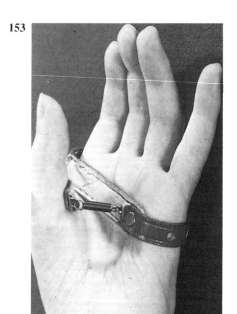

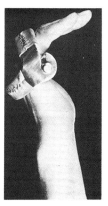

153 Two patients were supplied with splints for their hands.
(a) What are they called?
(b) What is their purpose?
(c) What is the difference between them?

154 The legs of a young man, born with considerable deformities.
(a) What abnormal features are apparent?
(b) What is the likely diagnosis?
(c) How may it be confirmed?

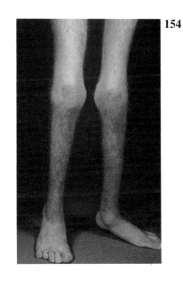

155 A woman with rheumatoid polyarthritis; both shoulders are badly affected. What does the arthrograph reveal?

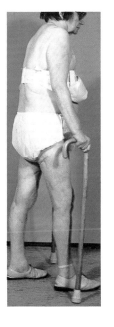

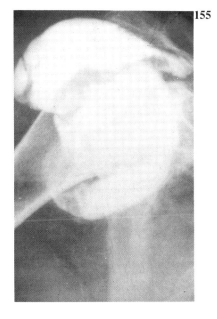

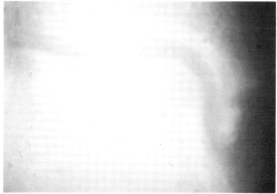

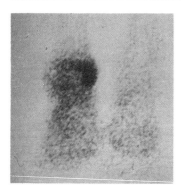

156 Several weeks after a young man fell down a flight of stairs he still had continuous pain on the medial aspect of his right ankle.
(a) What is the differential diagnosis?
(b) What simple tests would establish the diagnosis?

157 The patient complained of continuous aching in the arm.
(a) What is the probable diagnosis?
(b) How may it be tested?

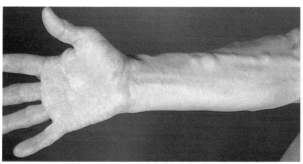

158 The deformed foot of a patient who had an attack of poliomyelitis in infancy.
(a) Define the deformity.
(b) Which muscles are affected?

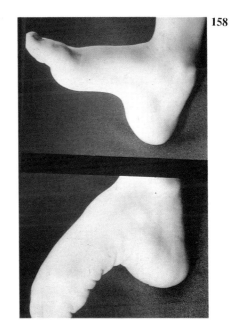

159 This patient's thumb was injured in a fall; there was swelling and pain at the base.
(a) By what eponym is this fracture known?
(b) What are its characteristics?

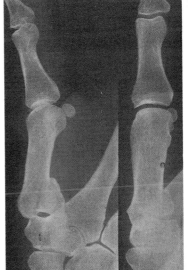

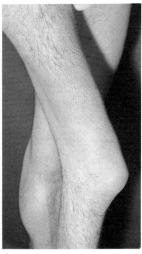

160 The right knee of a young man who suffered from poliomyelitis in infancy.
(a) What is this deformity and what are its elements?
(b) What has caused the deformity?

161 This boy's right shoulder frequently 'comes out of joint'. The radiograph showed only slight inferior subluxation of the glenohumeral joint.
(a) What is the probable diagnosis?
(b) How may it be established?

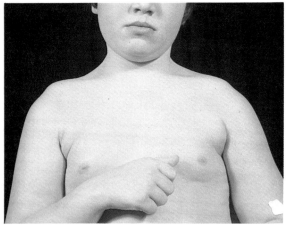

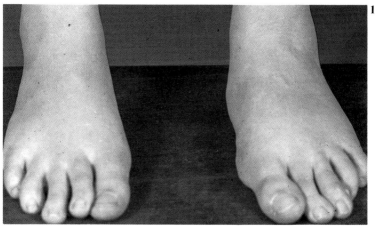

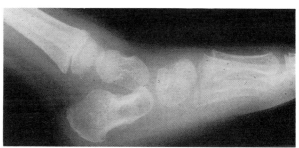

162 The patient complained of pain in the left foot.
(a) What is the deformity?
(b) What is the diagnosis?

163 Some weeks after a game of rugby a medical student presented with pain and swelling of his thigh; there were no clinical signs apart from measurable increase of girth and tenderness. What is the diagnosis?

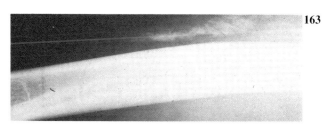

163

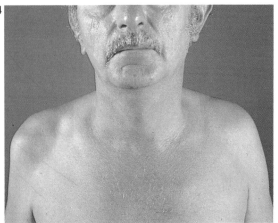

164 A 55-year-old man suddenly suffered intense pain in the right shoulder girdle which continued for several weeks; he is attempting to elevate both arms. Careful clinical examination revealed no sensory loss and the radiographs were normal.
(a) What is the diagnosis?
(b) Comment on the disorder.

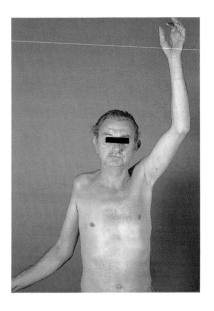

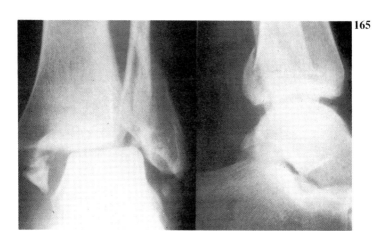

165 A woman slipped and damaged her right ankle, causing pain and swelling.
(a) What does the radiograph show?
(b) How do you classify this fracture and what is it eponymously called?

166 Radiograph of the wrist of a teenager, damaged in a fall. There is pain and deformity. What is the precise diagnosis?

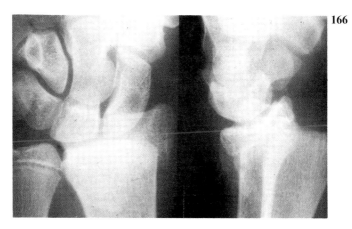

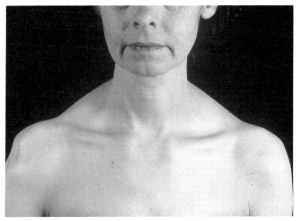

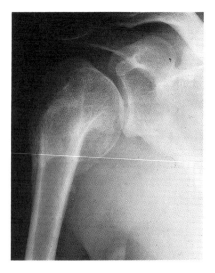

167 A middle-aged woman damaged her right shoulder some months before presenting.
(a) What is the condition?
(b) What is the differential diagnosis?
(c) How may it be established?

168 The foot of a patient whose leg was affected by poliomyelitis in infancy.
(a) What abnormality is shown?
(b) Which muscle is likely to have been paralysed?

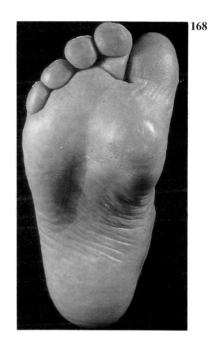

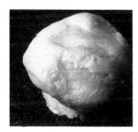

169 This patient had the head of her right radius removed at operation. What is the diagnosis?

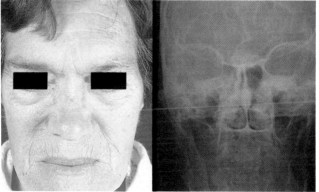

170

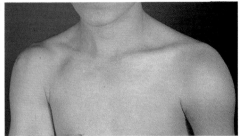

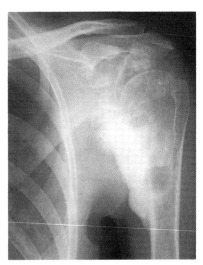

170 A 16-year-old boy has had a painful swelling of the left shoulder for 3 months; the diagnosis was established by biopsy and the photomicrograph is shown. What is the diagnosis?

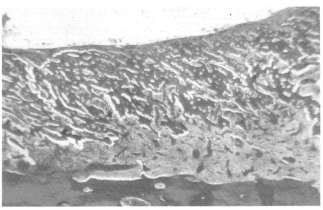

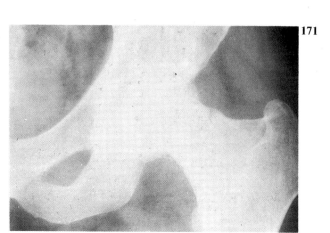

171 Radiograph of the left hip of an elderly woman who complained of pain in the groin and walked with a limp; she was not aware of having suffered any injury. What is the diagnosis?

172 This young man was concerned only about his appearance; he had no disability or pain. He was asked to contract his pectoral muscles by placing hands on hips. What is the abnormality?

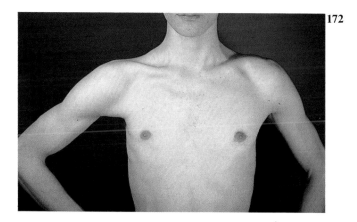

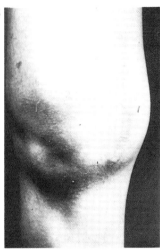

173 Swelling of the lower end of the femur and an effusion into the knee joint were found in a young man complaining of a painful knee.
(a) What is the diagnosis?
(b) What features assist diagnosis?

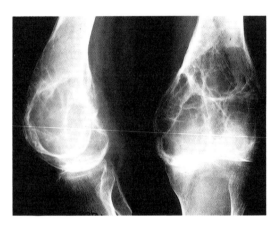

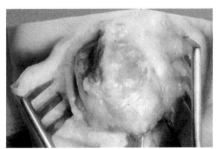

174 A young woman had a painless but tender swelling in the palm of her right hand; it was soft and semi-fluctuant. It is shown as at operation. What is it?

175 This child has disability associated with multiple deformities; in addition to those shown she has a moderately severe kyphoscoliosis and has had an operation for the repair of a cleft palate.
(a) Give a possible diagnosis.
(b) What is the most important investigation required for further management?

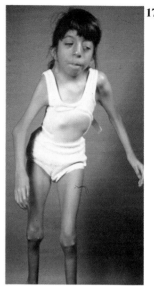

176 A young man had an injury causing pain on the top of the shoulder; he is asked to fold his arms across his chest.
(a) What inference can be made?
(b) What is the diagnosis?

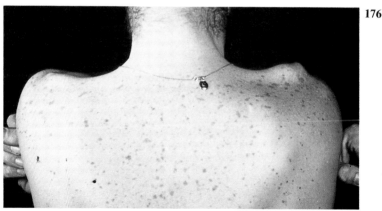

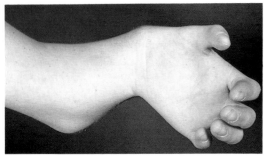

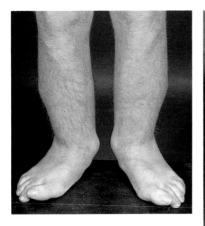

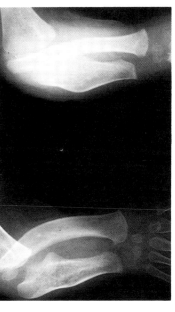

177 Severe deformities in an 18-year-old boy; his intelligence is entirely unimpaired.
(a) How would you classify this disorder?
(b) What is it called?

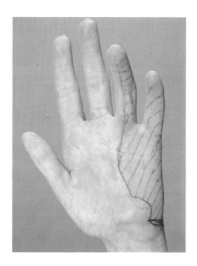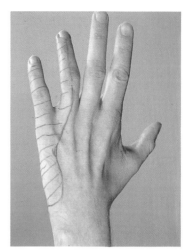

178 The hand of a patient who had a knife wound at the base of the palm; the marked area shows distribution of loss of sensibility of the skin.
(a) What other abnormal features are present?
(b) What is the diagnosis?

179 A swelling on the outer aspect of a young man's knee. What is the diagnosis?

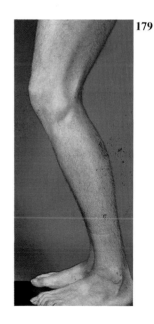

180

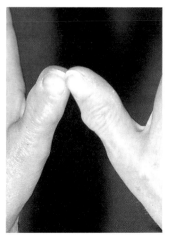 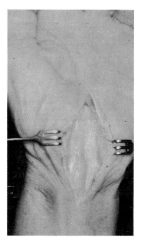

180 A 60-year-old woman had numbness and tingling in her left hand. At operation the median nerve was exposed.
(a) What sign is apparent in the clinical photograph?
(b) What is the swelling displayed at operation?
(c) What is the diagnosis?
(d) What are the symptoms and signs of this condition?

181

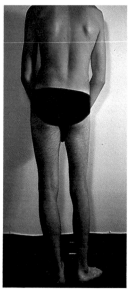

181 A young man complains of backache when he stands for any length of time; his spine is fully mobile and the radiographs are entirely normal.
(a) What may be the cause of the curvature?
(b) How may the diagnosis be tested?

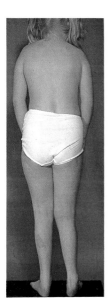
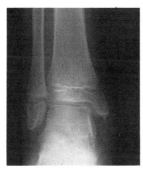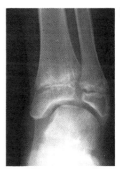

182 A girl with a short and underdeveloped right leg walks with a limp. Radiographs of her ankles are shown.
(a) What is this condition of the ankle joint?
(b) With what may it be associated?

183 Five years previously a young man had severe illness requiring drainage of pus from the knee; he now presents with limitation of extension of the knee.
(a) What is the most likely diagnosis?
(b) To what may the limitation of movement be attributed?

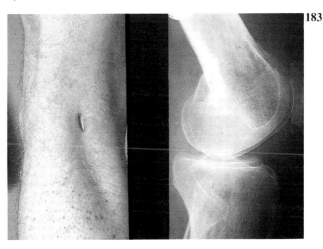

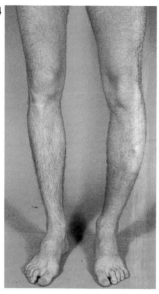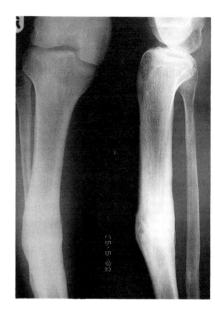

184 Five years after a motorcycle accident this young man presented with a deformed left leg. What is the nature of the *precise* deformity?

185 This patient suffered a crushing injury of her middle finger which was subsequently amputated. As pain continued, it was eventually disarticulated at the metacarpophalangeal joint. The nodule proximal to the amputation scar is very tender, and pressure caused unbearable pain. The patient feels as though she still has her finger. What is the diagnosis?

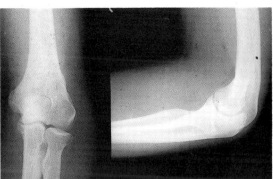

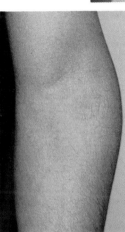

186 A teenager had fractured his elbow at 8 years of age.
(a) What is the deformity?
(b) What are its elements?

187 A middle-aged woman has a painful wrist.
(a) What is the diagnosis and what is it eponymously called?
(b) What sign most accurately confirms the diagnosis?

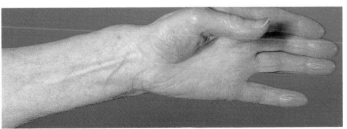

187

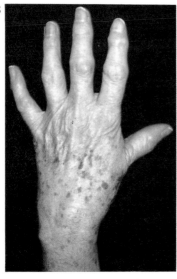

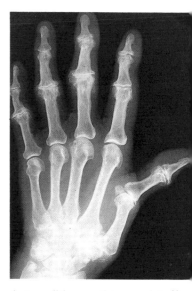

188 What are the swellings and with what condition are they associated?

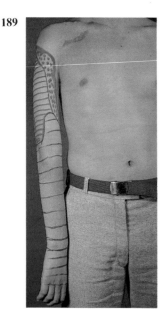

189 This young man was involved in a motorcycle accident; note the position of his arm and hand. The markings indicate: red dots — hypersensitivity; red lines — partial loss of sensibility; black lines — total loss of sensibility.
(a) What is the diagnosis?
(b) Precisely what damage has occurred?

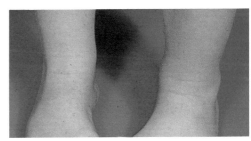

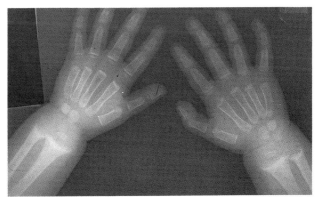

190 The ankles and wrists of a 6-year-old child who presented with swelling of these joints.
(a) What is the diagnosis?
(b) How may its aetiology be defined?

191 (a) What is the name and nature of this shoulder swelling?
(b) To what may it be attributed?

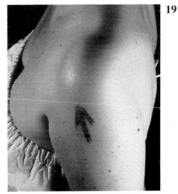

ANSWERS

[see page XXX] **indicates an illustration of that answer.**

1 (a) Postural forefoot varus; the bow legs are secondary to this deformity.
(b) Various types of rickets; tibia vara.

2 (a) Rheumatoid arthritis; the radiograph shows an advanced stage of the disease but is otherwise entirely typical.
(b) A rheumatoid nodule. (There is a similar nodule in the prepatellar region of her knee.)

3 Old compression fracture of the os calcis. *[see page 125]*

4 (a) Scleroderma.
(b) Open formal biopsy is essential to establish the diagnosis of a rare soft-tissue lesion of this type.

5 (a) 'Swan-neck' deformity of the fingers.
(b) Results from rupture of the sublimis tendon and associated disruption of the volar plates of the proximal interphalangeal joints.

6 (a) Bilateral recurrent subluxation of the patellae.
(b) Malalignment of the extensor quadriceps apparatus, demonstrated by measuring the q-angle. When this angle is increased beyond the normal average of 15° there is a tendency for the patellae to subluxate outwards when the knee is flexed.
(c) The q-angle is the angle between the line of pull of the quadriceps muscle from the anterior superior iliac spine to the top of the patella and line of the patellar ligament; q-angle refers to the quadriceps angle.

7 (a) Idiopathic congenital bowing of the tibia.
(b) Birth fracture; neurofibromatosis.

8 (a) Paget's disease of the tibia (diagnosis can be made without biopsy).
(b) The fibula is unaffected and hence a relative increase in the length of the tibia leads to its bowing.

9 (a) Congenital curly little toes; the condition has a very high familial incidence.
(b) Digitus minimus quintus varus.

10 Spina bifida occulta in the lumbosacral region and Sprengel deformity of the shoulder. The two conditions are possibly related.

11 (a) Obstetric paralysis — Klumpke type.
(b) The deformity is due to the normal action of muscles in the presence of paralysis of the muscles supplied by the damaged lower cords of the brachial plexus (C7/8 and T1), (see **38**).

12 (a) Metatarsus primus varus, possibly the commonest cause of hallux valgus and bunions.
(b) As in this patient, it may be developmental and familial.
(c) Classically, 'an inflamed adventitious bursa'. Its most common site is over the medial aspect of the prominent metatarsal head, often with related exostosis (see **42**).

13 Femoral nerve. The delineated area shows the sensory supply of the femoral nerve, including the prepatellar branch of its saphenous branch, and the distal sensory supply of the saphenous nerve. The tumour was a schwannoma of the femoral nerve.

14 Ankylosis of the right hip in severe adduction-flexion deformity. The patient keeps the left knee flexed to compensate for the relative shortening of the right leg.

15 (a) Volkmann's sign.
(b) Usually due to the contracture of ischaemic flexor muscles. In this case it is — unusually — due to a Baker's cyst emanating from the elbow and so displacing and stretching the forearm flexor muscles. *[see page 125]*

16 (a) Spondylolisthesis. The pattern is that of a dysplastic spondylolisthesis.
(b) The radiograph shows a very marked slip of L5 on S1. *[see page 125]*

17 Malunion of the mid-shaft of the left femur.

18 (a) Onycholysis due to Benoxaprofen therapy.
(b) Because of widespread complications, this drug has largely been discontinued.

19 (a) Rheumatoid polyarthritis; the wrist joint is severely affected.
(b) A mild but typical 'swan-neck' deformity.
(c) Rupture of the flexor sublimis at the wrist and simultaneous stretching of the interphalangeal joint capsule.

20 Synovial chondromatosis. The glenohumeral joint is very rarely affected by disease other than rheumatoid arthritis.

21 Simple carpal ganglion; there is virtually no differential diagnosis.

22 (a) Mild congenital deformation of the ribcage; a common anomaly of no consequence other than a minor aesthetic blemish.
(b) No treatment required, other than a full explanation of its benign nature.

23 Ainhum's disease; the Yoruba name for this affliction of the toe, the aetiology of which has not been established, but is possibly parasitic.

24 Necrobiosis lipodica. The patient being a known severe diabetic provided the diagnostic clue to this rare condition. Radiographs were normal.

25 Neurilemmoma. The diagnosis of multiple schwannomata was established by biopsy of the lesions in this rare case; the radiograph shows an extrapulmonary but intrapleural schwannoma.

26 (a) Scoliosis.
(b) Full forward flexion will show whether or not further investigation is required; in this patient the curvature did *not* disappear on full forward flexion (cf. postural scoliosis).

27 (a) Thomas' test.
(b) An important clinical method of determining hidden hip flexion. The lumbar lordosis is obliterated by flexing the opposite hip fully; the figure shows 70° fixed flexion deformity in the right hip.

28 (a) Generalised degenerative arthritis in all components of the glenohumeral and subacromial joints.
(b) 'Silent' rupture of the tendon of long head of biceps, a sign of glenohumeral arthropathy.

29 (a) Fibrous dysplasia of ulna; a non-malignant disorder of bone.
(b) Local excision and bone graft.

30 (a) Lambrinudi-type triple arthrodesis of the foot.
(b) Post-paralytic drop-foot. The joints distal to the ankle are excised and arthrodesed to correct the drop-foot; the ankle is left alone.

31 (a) Anterior drawer sign. This patient was able to demonstrate the instability himself — usually the sign must be elicited by the examining surgeon.
(b)Rupture of the anterior cruciate ligament and associated joint capsule.

32 (a) Dupuytren's contracture of the palmar fascia.
(b) An accurate family history often provides the clue to diagnosis.

33 Trevor's disease; a rare condition of tarso-epiphyseal aclasis, a congenital error of development affecting one or other side of the ankle, knee or wrist.

34 Soft tissue constriction at the site of the bandage and — more importantly — gross wastage of the muscles below due to ischaemic contracture; the skin of the foot is also ischaemic.

35 (a) Spondylo-epiphyseal dysostosis.
(b) All forms of dwarfism, in particular the Brailsford-Morquio syndrome with its characteristic vertebral shape.
(c) A radiograph of the spine or routine skeletal survey; analysis of mucopolysaccharide excretion in the urine (see **51**)

36 (a) Juvenile kyphosis (Scheuermann's disease).
(b) It may simulate tuberculosis of the spine.
(c) When in doubt, a blood sedimentation rate (ESR) should be done.

37 (a) Congenital talipes equinovarus; treatment has been unsatisfactory and the heel remains in equinus and inversion.
(b) An elongation of the tendo Achillis, so that the heel can get fully to the ground.

38 (a) Obstetric paralysis — Erb's palsy.
(b) A form of birth paralysis of the arm due to injury of the brachial plexus. In Erb's palsy the upper cords of the plexus (C5/6/7) are affected; the deformity is brought about by the action of the *un*paralysed pronator/flexor group of muscles of the arm and forearm (see **11**).

39 Congenital osteogenic scoliosis. *[see page 125]*

40 (a) Outward rotation deformity; the radiographs are spurious.
(b) Only clinical examination provides the correct answer. *[see page 127]*

41 (a) Congenital arterio-venous intramuscular malformation; at operation the entire muscle mass of the flexor-pronator group was affected by angiomatous infiltration.
(b) Arterio-venous aneurysm; angiosarcoma; myosarcoma.
(c) The diagnosis was established by arteriography. *[see page 125]*

42 (a) A 'bunionette'.
(b) An adventitious bursa overlying an exostosis on the prominent head of the 5th metatarsal (see **12**).

43 Paralytic scoliosis; it used to be seen frequently following anterior poliomyelitis.

44 (a) Post-traumatic genu varum.
(b) An old rupture of the anterior cruciate and internal lateral ligaments.

45 Division of the terminal sensory branch of the radial nerve (iatrogenic); the nerve must be carefully retracted during operation for de Quervain's disease.

46 (a) Genu recurvatum.
(b) The deformity in this case developed due to premature epiphyseal fusion of the anterior part of the upper tibial growth plate at an operation for recurrent dislocation of the patella; the operation must not be done before epiphyseal maturity (see **49**).

47 (a) Os tibialis externum.
(b) One of the several congenital embryonic ossicles found frequently around the ankle and hindfoot.

48 (a) Internal tibial torsion.
(b) None required; the condition will correct itself.

49 (a) Genu recurvatum.
(b) In this case the deformity is due to old disruption of the posterior cruciate ligament and capsule of the right knee causing postero-lateral instability of the joint (see **46**).

50 (a) Clawed toes.
(b) Neurological investigation of the lower limbs; when in doubt, a radiograph of the lumbar spine should be requested to confirm that toe-clawing is not a symptom of neurological disorder.

51 (a) Brailsford-Morquio syndrome.
(b) Thought to be due to an abnormality of mucopolysaccharide IV excretion (see **35**).

52 (a) Pes plano valgus.
(b) For accurate diagnosis it is essential to know whether or not the deformity can be passively corrected.

53 (a) Nutritional rickets; the appearance of the widened growth plates at the wrist is diagnostic.
(b) The cause of the rickets must be determined by clinical and laboratory investigation.

54 (a) Multilocular ganglion arising from the peroneal tendon sheath.
(b) The dumb-bell shape arises because its centre is compressed by the peroneal retinaculum.

55 (a) The back is held stiffly with obliteration of the normal lumbar lordosis.
(b) Straight-leg-raising on the right is limited; it is less than 20° in this patient, at which point there is severe pain down the leg.
(c) The signs strongly suggest intervertebral disc protrusion with pressure on L5 or S1 nerve roots. *[see page 126]*
(d) Myelography is essential.

56 Left sciatic nerve injury associated with a comminuted fracture of the pelvis. Careful scrutiny shows muscle wasting of the whole left lower limb. The sensory component of the medial popliteal nerve was involved, as well as both sensory and motor components of the lateral popliteal nerve.

57 (a) Pigmented villonodular synovitis.
(b) By excision biopsy, although careful scrutiny of the radiograph shows a small lytic lesion on the articular surface of the patella, typical in appearance.

58 Psoriatic arthropathy.

59 (a) Acromegaly.
(b) Polyarthritis; carpal tunnel syndrome.

60 (a) Klippel-Feil syndrome.
(b) Osteogenic type of scoliosis, as seen on the radiograph; elevation of the right scapula; low hairline.

61 (a) Acute gonococcal septic arthritis.
(b) By examination of the aspirate.

62 Rheumatoid polyarthritis; soft tissue nodules arising from tendons and joints are common in rheumatoid disease (see **19**).

63 (a) Pes cavo varus.
(b) The majority of cases are neurogenic in origin.
(c) Radiography of the lumbar spine is obligatory to demonstrate any congenital abnormality, such as spina bifida at the lumbosacral level. *[see page 126]*

64 (a) Genu valgum; developmental (idiopathic) knock-knees.
(b) The condition almost inevitably corrects itself providing there is no associated disease or skeletal abnormality; the treatment is entirely expectant and reassuring.

65 (a) Ischaemic contracture of calf muscles associated with a fractured tibia; this occurs much more commonly than is generally supposed.
(b) The marks of transfixion pins in the upper and lower tibia and the healed fracture of midshaft tibia and fibula.

66 'Lobster-claw' deformity; a congenital deformity seen in the toes of both feet, the right foot showing the fully developed deformation.

67 (a) Pseudarthrosis — ununited fracture of the shaft of the tibia and fibula; the radiograph shows hypertrophic callus at the site of pseudarthrosis.
(b) The multiple scarring is indicative of several previous failed operations and, probably, infection. Almost certainly this injury was caused by direct violence, and several unsuccessful attempts have been made to achieve union.

68 (a) Hallux flexus; a somewhat archaic term found in old orthopaedic literature to describe the deformity of the big toe which can be due to a variety of causes.
(b) In this case the deformity is due to the action of surviving intrinsic musculature to the big toe in the presence of paralysis of the antagonists, extensor brevis and longus. (Note that deformity is *not* caused by paralysed muscle.)

69 (a) Trendelenburg's sign.
(b) Indicates instability of the hip joint; stability of the hip relied on the integrity of the abductor muscles and an efficient hip joint.

70 (a) 'Pigeon-toe' gait is a transient postural abnormality frequently seen in children, caused by persistent foetal alignment of the hips.
(b) Reassurance that the condition invariably corrects itself.

71 Hallux valgus and multiple pressure points on all the toes. On the right foot there is a typical bunion (adventitious bursa overlying an exostosis on the head of the medial aspect of the first metatarsal). The second toe overrides the big toe; deformity is caused by a subluxation or dislocation of the 2nd metatarsophalangeal joint — a common complication of hallux valgus.

72 Internal rotational deformity which cannot be seen on a standard radiograph. Clinical examination is essential and shows that there is a marked internal rotation deformity of the right leg. *[see page 126]*

73 Recurrent dislocation of the patella. *[see page 127]*

74 (a) Bilateral congenital radial club hands.
(b) Marked radial deviation at the wrist; absence or underdevelopment of the radius (the single forearm bone on the radiograph is the ulna); comparative increase in the size of the ulnar fingers.

75 (a) Intrinsic muscle wasting with 'guttering' of the back of the hand.
(b) Wasting of this kind, from any cause, most commonly occurs secondary to ulnar nerve lesion.

76 Poland's syndrome; microsyndactyly of one hand with absence of the costal part of the pectoralis major muscle on the same side.

77 Post-measles encephalopathy; in this case the pes cavus was secondary to measles encephalitis in infancy. The condition is bilateral and symmetrical. The spasticity indicates an upper motor neuron lesion, therefore the pathology must lie above the level of the spinal cord supplying these muscles, i.e. above the lumbosacral level, involving either the pyramidal tract or the brain.

78 (a) Ollier's disease, (enchondromatosis, dyschondroplasia).
(b) Disparity in the growth of the arms.

79 (a) Accessory nerve palsy. The trapezius muscle has been paralysed as a result of division of the accessory nerve at an operation to remove cervical lymph nodes.

80 Colloidal gold; a rash occasionally develops when this has been used for treatment of rheumatoid arthritis.

81 (a) The commonest cause of a neuropathic pressure ulcer is diabetes; other causes are any form of peripheral neuropathy or peripheral vascular disease.
(b) Immediate testing for diabetes.

82 (a) Sudeck's atrophy.
(b) The very shiny skin on the back of the hand; marked osteoporosis of the carpal bones.

83 (a) 'Wind-swept' deformity with genu varum on the right leg and genu valgum on the left.
(b) The principal site of deformation is on the metaphyseal side of the growth plate.
(c) Metaphyseal dysostosis, of the Schmid type, which is relatively benign.

84 Rupture of the rotator cuff of the shoulder; loss of active outward rotation is one characteristic sign.

85 (a) Gouty arthritis with tophus.
(b) The most important investigation is a serum acid estimation, preferably carried out during an acute phase of the disease.

86 (a) Brachial plexus injury involving the lower cord (C8/T1).
(b) The enophthalmos and constricted pupil is a Horner's syndrome caused by damage of the cervical sympathetic trunk carried in the lower cord of the brachial plexus.

87 (a) Klippel-Feil syndrome; The combination of thoracic deformity, high shoulder and gross abnormality of ossification of the cervical and upper dorsal vertebrae is typical (see **60**).
(b) No treatment is indicated unless the deformity is very severe.

88 Head tilted to the left, chin upwards and to the right; right eye higher than the left; left sternomastoid muscle more prominent than the right; clinical examination showed she was unable to turn her head fully to the left, but could do so to the right. The diagnosis is torticollis (wry neck).

89 (a) Lacertus fibrosus; an aponeurotic band from the biceps tendon to the fascia of the forearm.
(b) There is no clinical significance and no treatment is required.

90 (a) Ehlers-Danlos syndrome.
(b) The feet show chronic pseudotumours of the skin in the neighbourhood of the joints — part of the original description of the syndrome; there is also cutis hyperelastica and dermatolysis.
(c) The same pathology occasionally occurs in the elastic tissue of large arteries, causing an aneurysm.

91 (a) Spondylolisthesis.
(b) The spondylolitic pattern on the radiograph shows the body of the 5th lumbar vertebra displaced forwards by more than half its width on the body of the 1st sacral vertebra; the paravertebral joints are completely disrupted.
[see page 127]

92 (a) Venous angioma of the sole of the foot.
(b) If the foot is elevated the swellings can be virtually emptied; the application of a venous constricting cuff at the ankle will cause them rapidly to increase in size.

93 (a) Baker's cyst. A synovial protrusion from the knee deeply into the calf, originally described as arising from tuberculosis of the knee joint.
(b) Nowadays more commonly seen as a consequence of rheumatoid arthritis.
(c) Gross destructive arthropathy.

94 Congenital radio-ulnar synostosis; discrepancy in bone length is associated with arrest of growth at the upper radial epiphysis.

95 (a) Congenital talipes equinovarus.
(b) 'Club foot'.
(c) The word 'talipes' is a combination of the Latin 'talus' ankle and 'pes' foot; any deformity of the foot is called 'talipes' followed by the type of deformity. In this case the foot is in equinus and the forefoot turned inwards in varus = talipes equinovarus.

96 (a) Infected pseudarthrosis.
(b) Incisions over the tibia and marks of at least two sinus tracks can be seen. The radiograph shows not only the pseudarthrosis with some hypertrophic callus, but two screws in situ. There has clearly been a fracture of the right tibia and fibula in which attempts at stabilisation have failed, infection has supervened, followed by pseudarthrosis (see **67**).

97 (a) Ulnar drift.
(b) Due to the line of pull of the long muscles to the fingers, with simultaneous weakening and destruction of the collateral ligaments of the metacarpophalangeal joints, the hands may characteristically drift ulnarwards.

98 (a) Madelung's deformity.
(b) A congenital deformity, possibly due to injury of the lower radial growth plate leading to differential growth of radius and ulna whereby the hand is displaced and the lower end of ulna, being the longer, becomes more apparent. It is occasionally seen as part of a generalised skeletal dysplasia.

99 (a) Considerable alteration in the shape of the calf muscles on the right side with marked underdevelopment. Both feet are abnormal and deformed: on the left the forefoot is adducted so that the big toe can be clearly seen to peep out past the heel; the right foot shows the opposite deformity, ie the foot is severely turned outwards and fully pronated, so that the little toe is more evident on the outer side.
(b) Arthrogryposis multiplex congenita.
(c) Radiograph of both lower limbs, to show absence of normal muscle compartments; biopsy of the more obviously affected muscles, to show replacement of normal muscle fibres by non-specific fibroblastic tissue.

100 Osteogenic scoliosis; in this patient it was secondary to a hemivertebra, seen in the radiograph just above T12.

101 'Subacromial painful arc', caused by some impingement or lesion of the rotator cuff or subacromial bursa.

102 (a) Scheuermann's disease, osteochondritis juvenalis of the spine.
(b) It occasionally affects the lumbar spine, as in this case, when it may be confused with tuberculosis.
(c) Appropriate serological investigations are essential (see **36**).

103 (a) Early Dupuytren's contracture.
(b) There is frequently a family history; the other hand and soles of both feet must be carefully examined for evidence of the disease (see **138**).

104 (a) The ossification centre of the left femoral head is slightly under-developed and stands proud of the acetabulum as compared to the right side.
(b) Progress is entirely satisfactory.
(c) Further immobilisation in splints is mandatory.

105 (a) Congenital absence of clavicular part of right pectoralis major.
(b) The patient is asked to contract both pectoral muscles by placing hands on hips and pressing firmly; the defect then becomes obvious. (Congenital absence of part or whole of one or more muscles is well documented.)

106 Pseudarthrosis probably associated with neurofibromatosis. Both bones of the forearm are affected to different degrees, causing dislocation of the head of the radius during growth. As there was no history of a single major accident, and because the condition had been modified by several surgical interventions, the diagnosis is not certain, but is thought to be due to neurofibromatosis.

107 (a) The skin of the hand is bluish and atrophic; marked wasting of all the small muscles particularly the interossei, indicating damage to the ulnar nerve; wasting of the thenar muscles (pulp of the thumb) indicative of damage to the median nerve; widespread loss of sensibility of all digits.
(b) Longstanding complete paralysis due to low division of median and ulnar nerves in the forearm; that the long flexor muscles to the fingers have survived indicates that the lesion was below the level of their innervation; typical end-result of an untreated 'cut-wrist'.

108 (a) Marked lumbar scoliosis; tilting of the pelvis causing relative shortening of the left leg; marked retraction and clawing of all the toes of the left foot (on which a surgical scar can be seen); slight inversion of the left heel.
(b) In addition to a slight angled curvature there is obvious deficiency of the bony elements and a very wide distance between the pedicles.
(c) Spinal dysraphism; frequently associated with a lower motor neuron lesion affecting one or more nerve roots.

109 Malunited fracture of the proximal phalanx of the little finger. Angulation at site of fracture has occurred at the extreme end of the proximal phalanx so that the long arm of the distal fragment has caused a proportionally greater deformity than would be expected from such a trivial fracture. Fractures at the ends of long bones are more likely to cause deformity than similar fractures towards the centre of the bone.

110 (a) Teratogenic agent.
(b) Complete examination of the child; in this case the deformity of the foot had an entirely different pattern from that of the hand. Multiple congenital abnormalities suggest that the infant was subject to a teratogenic influence in utero, such as the drug thalidomide.

111 (a) Volkmann's sign, produced because the flexor muscles are relatively short so that they allow the fingers to be straight only when the wrist is fully flexed; when the wrist is extended the shortened muscles cause passive finger flexion.
(b) Ischaemic contracture of the long flexor muscles of the fingers caused by damage to the muscle belly in the forearm.

112 (a) Although there is a very slight scoliosis when he stands erect, he should be examined in the flexed, toe-touching position to determine whether the scoliosis has a rotational element; in full forward flexion there is no rotation and the curve straightens out.
(b) Postural scoliosis.

113 Osteoid osteoma of L4 pedicle. The lumbar myelography, performed to exclude an intervertebral disc rupture or a spinal tumour, revealed no lesion (see **156**).

114 'Cuff arthropathy'; the head of the humerus shows hyperaemia and erosion of the articular cartilage.

115 (a) Hypophosphataemic rickets.
(b) Type of rickets must be determined by comprehensive serological investigations, especially renal function tests; this patient showed constant low levels of serum phosphorus due to renal tubular dysfunction.

116 (a) Rheumatoid polyarthritis.
(b) Blood-sedimentation rate (ESR); Rose-Waller and latex tests. In this patient the ESR was 65 and the other tests strongly positive.

117 (a) Prader-Willi syndrome; scoliosis is a common accompaniment of the obesity, usually resistant to diet.
(b) It is essential that the child is fully investigated for thyroid and other endocrine dysfunction before making this rare diagnosis.

118 (a) Subcutaneous lipoma.
(b) Shows characteristic translucency of the tumour.
(c) Infrapatellar bursitis; a soft tissue tumour.

119 Acute anterior dislocation of the sternoclavicular joint.

120 (a) Extreme pes valgus (post-traumatic).
(b) Tibialis anterior and posterior completely erased while peroneal muscles were undamaged and continued to act normally, in the absence of their antagonists.

121 (a) 'Signal-arm' prosthesis.
(b) Pathological fractures of the subtrochanteric region of the femur.

122 The fracture of the middle phalanx of the middle finger has healed with rotational deformity.

123 (a) Cyst of the lateral meniscus; virtually the only swelling on the outer side of the knee-joint appearing in exactly this position and most prominent at 30° of flexion (see **179**).
(b) A lipoma; a ganglion from the superior tibiofibular joint.

124 The left foot is slightly cavus and the right slightly valgus. Differences in the shape of the feet can have serious implications; in this case the diagnosis was spinal dysraphism. *[see page 127]*

125 Malunion of fractured tibia; the appearance somewhat mimics that seen in Paget's disease of the tibia. *[see page 127]*

126 (a) Pes cavus and clawed toes.
(b) Spinal radiograph mandatory. In this case there is spina bifida of L4 with considerable laminar defect; a high proportion of patients with pes cavus have a causative neurological abnormality. *[see page 127]*

127 Investigation of the urine for mucopolysaccharide excretion; lateral radiograph of the skull may be useful, as in this case of mucopolysaccharidosis (MPS IV), to show very tiny pituitary fossae. *[see page 128]*

128 (a) Ankylosing spondylitis; severe limitation of spinal movements associated with obliteration of the sacro-iliac joints (see radiograph) are characteristic.
(b) Blood sedimentation rate (invariably raised when the disease is active); estimation of the HLA (commonly raised).

129 Lisfranc fracture; fracture-dislocation through the tarsometatarsal level (Lisfranc's joint); often reduces itself or is easily reduced under manipulation, but leaves damage which subsequently becomes evident.

130 (a) Anterolateral curvature of the shaft of right tibia, implying a defect of the fibula.
(b) Just above the iliac crest, one — or possibly two — café-au-lait patches can be seen, suggesting the diagnosis of neurofibromatosis.
(c) Variable: the usual form of anterolateral bowed tibia has an excellent prognosis, but when associated with neurofibromatosis the prognosis should be guarded. *[see page 128]*

131 Osgood-Schlatter disease; although a radiograph is hardly necessary, fragments of bone can be seen as soon as the fragmented tibial tubercle becomes ossified.

132 (a) Severe wasting of the first dorsal interosseous muscle of the left hand.
(b) Gradual compression of the ulnar nerve at the elbow (see **152**).

133 Gorham's disease; massive osteolysis, or vanishing-bone disease; only rarely occurs in the clavicle.

134 Osteochondritis dissecans of the lateral condyle of the femur, the site most commonly affected. Changes range from simple shedding of the overlying articular cartilage to complete collapse of the condyle; classically a loose body is shed into the joint, but not always.

135 'Bucket-handle' tear; of the many patterns of rupture of the meniscus, this is typical of a ruptured lateral meniscus.

136 (a) Familial idiopathic genu valgum.
(b) In a unilateral case, follow-up is essential.
(c) The inter-malleolar distance, measured standing with legs extended.

137 (a) Froment's test.
(b) Weakness or paralysis of flexor pollicis brevis and impairment of conduction of the median nerve supplying muscles of the thenar eminence.
(c) In attempting to grasp the card between the thumb and base of index finger, flexor pollicis longus takes over from the weakened pollicis brevis, so that the thumb collapses into flexion at the interphalangeal joint.

138 Dupuytren's contracture; the pathological process which produced contracture of the palmar fascia is occasionally seen in the feet; it does not cause contracture of the toes because of the anatomical disposition of the plantar fascia compared with the palmar fascia (see **103**).

139 Hammer-toes and digitus minimus quintus varus. Both congenital deformities are familial and must be distinguished from clawed toes.

140 (a) Posterior dislocation of the shoulder.
(b) A true lateral radiograph accurately depicts the diagnosis.

141 (a) Unable either to extend or flex the terminal interphalangeal joint.
(b) Trapped extensor apparatus of the little finger.

142 (a) Charcot's shoulder joint; neuropathic arthropathy due to syringo-myelia. Note the speed of destruction which has developed in the short period of six months in the left glenohumeral joint.
(b) Clinical neurological examination of the left hand shows typical dissociation of sensory loss.

143 (a) Persistent foetal alignment of the femoral neck.
(b) 'Squinting patellae' is a transient postural anomaly associated with persistent anteversion of the femoral necks.

144 (a) Normal movement of the ankle associated with no movement whatever in the hindfoot at the subtaloid joint, ie no inversion or eversion.
(b) Calcaneonavicular bar, one type of congenital tarsal coalition.

145 (a) Mucopolysaccharidosis; one form of generalised musculoskeletal disease produced by the abnormal metabolism of MPS IV; it has a number of slightly different clinical manifestations. Type IV (as in this case) also being known as Morquio's disease.
(b) Blood and urine analyses for abnormal mucopolysaccharide excretion; a skeletal survey because all growth-plates will be affected.

146 (a) Proximal femoral focal deficiency.
(b) This disorder ranges from congenital coxa vara, in its mildest form, to almost complete absence of the femoral shaft, as in this patient.

147 Careful examination of the photograph reveals a tiny café-au-lait patch above the crest of the left ilium, indicative of neurofibromatosis.

148 (a) Supracondylar spur of the humerus.
(b) Attached to the tip of the spur is the rudimentary ligament of Struthers with the median nerve and a branch of the brachial artery passing beneath it; the artery may become obstructed. *[see page 128]*

149 Inclusion dermoid cyst.

150 (a) Schwannoma (neurilemmona).
(b) Usually not malignant, it interferes with neural conduction only by internal pressure; can be completely shelled out from within the nerve sheath.

151 (a) Adolescent coxa vara, slipped upper femoral epiphysis.
(b) An irritable hip, combined with loss of extremes of internal rotation and flexion.
(c) Secondary degenerative arthritis and deformation of the femoral head due to interference of its blood supply have already become established.

152 (a) Wasting of the interossei muscles.
(b) Tardy ulnar palsy caused by impairment of conduction of the ulnar nerve at the elbow, in this case by trapping of the nerve as it enters the tunnel between the two heads of flexor carpi ulnaris.
(c) 'Tardy' because it develops gradually (see **132**).

153 (a) A 'knuckle-duster' splints.
(b) They can be used to replace the action of temporarily paralysed interossei following ulnar nerve injury.
(c) The picture on the right combines the knuckle-duster with a device for maintaining palmar abduction of the thumb; this is used to replace paralysis of all the intrinsic musculature in a combined median and ulnar nerve lesion.

154 (a) Both legs thin and spindly, due to absence of contractile muscle tissue; knees flexed; left foot shows severe planovalgus.
(b) Arthrogryposis multiplex congenita.
(c) Confirmation rarely necessary; a radiograph will show characteristic absence of normal muscle compartments, a biopsy will show absence of normal muscle tissue.

155 Rupture of the rotator cuff; the contrast medium spreads from the glenohumeral joint into the subacromial bursa through the defective cuff.

156 (a) Osteoid osteoma of the medial malleolus, to be differentiated from an ununited fracture at the tip of the medial malleolus.
(b) The only test worth a trial is use of aspirin in large doses for short time, which characteristically relieves the pain of an osteoid osteoma.

157 (a) Congenital venous angiomata due to absence of valves.
(b) By venography or by simply applying a venous tourniquet to the upper arm.

158 (a) Pes calcaneocavus.
(b) Completely paralysed calf muscle; its antagonists have survived to produce the deformity.

159 (a) Bennett's fracture.
(b) Fracture at the base of the 1st metacarpal bone is characteristically oblique with a degree of subluxation of the carpometacarpal joint.

160 (a) Triple deformity of the knee; the three elements are flexion, posterior subluxation and outward rotation.
(b) Relative imbalance of stronger lateral hamstrings, in the presence of paralysed medial hamstrings and weak quadriceps.

161 (a) Recurrent (habitual) posterior dislocation of the shoulder.
(b) By pentothal study; when given a small induction dose, the boy's shoulder immediately reduced into normal position but re-dislocated as he emerged from anaesthesia.

162 (a) Pes planovalgus; the radiograph shows its cause.
(b) Congenital vertical talus.

163 Frequently called 'myositis ossificans', it is an ossifying haematoma beneath vastus intermedius. Clinically it may present as 'a fractured femur without a fracture'.

164 Neuralgic amyotrophy, paralytic brachial neuritis. A not uncommon disorder; although principally of the shoulder girdle, other muscles may be affected; thought to be due to viral infection.

165 (a) Bimalleolar fracture-dislocation of the ankle.
(b) Although often classified as a second degree abduction/external rotation fracture (in general terms a Pott's fracture) it should be more clearly defined as a guide to treatment.

166 Separation of the lower radial growth-plate, Salter-Harris type II.

167 (a) Subluxation of the shoulder.
(b) Paralysis of the deltoid due to circumflex palsy.
(c) By the simple clinical test of isometric contraction of the deltoid; the patient is asked to abduct the shoulder while the arm is held to the side and if a contraction can be felt, deltoid is not paralysed.

168 (a) Depression of the first metatarsal head.
(b) Caused by normal action of peroneus lognus, unopposed by its paralysed antagonist, tibialis anterior.

169 Acromegalic arthropathy.

170 Parosteal osteosarcoma; one of the few malignant tumours of bone treatable by conservative resection.

171 Stress or fatigue fracture of the femoral neck; possibly precedes many cases of fractured neck of femur.

172 Congenital absence of clavicular portion of pectoralis major; a benign and not uncommon congenital abnormality related to Poland's syndrome (see **76**).

173 (a) Giant cell tumour.
(b) Typically positioned at the lower end of the femur and extending up to the articular margin.

174 Pigmented villonodular synovitis; blue-stained areas contain iron pigment, signifying haemorrhage.

175 (a) Turner's syndrome.
(b) Chromosome analysis and typing is essential to establish the diagnosis and for accurate genetic counselling to the family; the opinion of an educational psychologist is necessary for management of the child.

176 Dislocation of acromioclavicular joint; instability of this joint best revealed by forced adduction of the arms across the chest.

177 (a) A form of mesomelic dwarfism.
(b) Terminal agenesis.

178 (a) Wasting of small muscles of the hand, particularly dorsal interossei; slight clawing of ring and little fingers.
(b) Low division of the ulnar nerve.

179 Cyst of the lateral meniscus; the only swelling on the outer side of the knee which is maximal at about 30° flexion and becomes smaller on either side of the angle (see **123**).

180 (a) In competitive palmar abduction the right thumb is stronger than the left, causing the left to collapse.
(b) The swelling is usually called a neuroma, although it principally consists of oedematous fluid within the nerve sheath, proximal to its site of constriction.
(c) Carpal tunnel syndrome, involving compression of the median nerve by the transverse carpal ligament.
(d) Pain and tingling in the thumb and index finger, worse at night; clumsiness in handling small objects. Loss of power of palmar abduction of thumb; diminution of sensibility in the distribution of the median nerve to thumb and finger; a positive Tinel's sign at the wrist, immediately proximal to the carpal tunnel. The symptoms can often be reproduced, either by application of a venous tourniquet to the arm, or by flexing the wrist for several minutes.

181 (a) Postural scoliosis, due to unequal leg length.
(b) In this case, when standing with the right foot on a 5 cm block, the spinal curvature corrects itself.

182 (a) 'Ball-and-socket' ankle joint.
(b) Usually associated with other skeletal congenital abnormalities, such as fusion of joints distal to the ankle in tarsal coalition, as in this case of congenital hemiatrophy.

183 (a) Acute pyogenic arthritis, fully resolved by appropriate treatment; the radiographs are normal apart from doubtful mild osteoporosis.
(b) Persistent periarticular fibrosis.

184 The appearance of anterolateral angulation is spurious; the deformity is almost always rotational. The patient should be carefully examined for malrotation of the leg at the site of the fracture; in this patient there is an internal rotation deformity which can only be clinically evaluated (see **72**).

185 Phantom finger, amputation causalgia; at the base of the disarticulated finger is an amputation neuroma.

186 (a) 'Gunstock deformity' of the elbow.
(b) Due to a malunited supracondylar fracture, the deformity consists of several elements: varus, medial rotation, extension of the lower fragment.

187 (a) de Quervain's disease, stenosing tendovaginitis of APL and EPB.
(b) By putting the wrist into full ulnar deviation then depressing thumb into the palm to stretch affected tendon sheaths.

188 Heberden's nodes are swellings of the distal interphalangeal joints associated with osteoarthritis; in distinction from Bouchard's nodes which affect the proximal interphalangeal joints, swelling of which — as well as the metacarpophalangeal joints — is most frequently seen in rheumatoid arthritis.

189 (a) Traction injury to the brachial plexus — complete.
(b) All nerve roots beyond C5 damaged; sensory involvement C6/7/8/T1 inclusive. The arm lies flail to the side in internal rotation because of total muscle power loss beyond C5; its position is determined by the action of undamaged nerve supply to subscapularis, a strong internal rotator of the shoulder supplied by C5.

190 (a) Nutritional rickets.
(b) A careful history and analysis of the diet was sufficient, in this case, to establish the nature of the rickets.

191 (a) Subacromial bursitis.
(b) Any lesion affecting synovial tissue (eg rheumatoid arthritis) or in the subacromial joint (eg a cuff impingement or minor rupture).

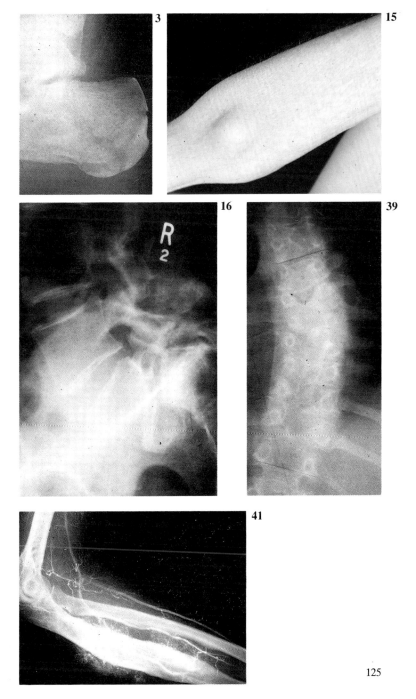

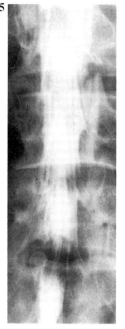

55

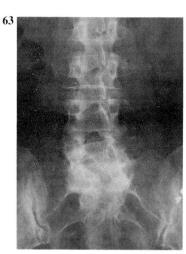

63

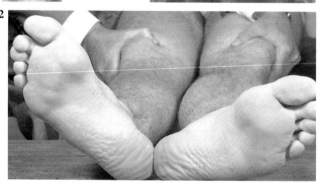

72

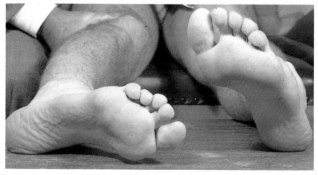

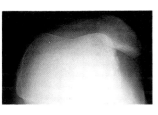

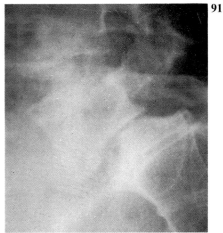

91

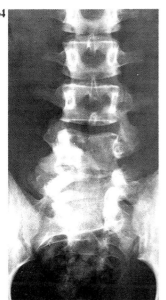

40 **125**

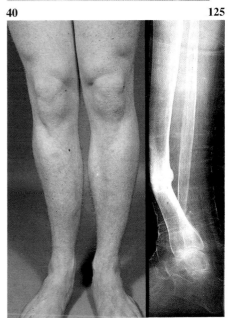

26

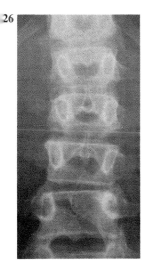

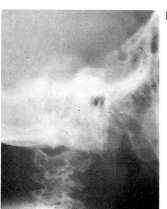

127

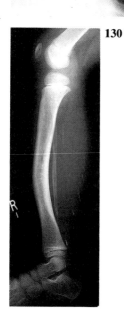

130

148